Paediatric Drug Handling

ULLA Postgraduate pharmacy series

Series Editors-in-Chief

Professor Alexander T Florence
CBE, DSc, FRSC, FRSE, FRPharmS
The School of Pharmacy, University of London, UK

Professor Anthony C Moffat
BPharm, PhD, DSc, CChem, FRSC, FRPharmS
The School of Pharmacy, University of London, UK

Other titles in the ULLA postgraduate pharmacy series include:
Pharmaceutical Toxicology
Paediatric Drug Handling
Molecular Biopharmaceutics
Proteomics and Metabolomics in Pharmaceutical Science
Biomedical and Pharmaceutical Polymers
International Pharmacy Practice Research

NB: some of titles listed are forthcoming/not yet published

Paediatric Drug Handling

Ian Costello
BPharm, MSc, MBA, MRPharmS
Deputy Chief Pharmacist
St George's Hospital
London, UK

Paul F Long
BSc, MSc, PhD
Senior Lecturer in Molecular Microbiology
Microbiology Group, Department of Pharmaceutics and Centre for
  Paediatric Pharmacy Research
The School of Pharmacy, University of London
London, UK

Ian K Wong
BSc, MSc, PhD, MRPharmS
Professor and Director of the Centre for Paediatric Pharmacy Research
The School of Pharmacy, University of London
London, UK

Catherine Tuleu
PhD, Docteur en Pharmacie, Cert Ed, MRPharmS
Lecturer in Pharmaceutics and Deputy Director at the Centre for
  Paediatric Pharmacy Research
The School of Pharmacy, University of London
London, UK

Vincent Yeung
PhD, MBA, MRPharmS
GCP Inspector
Medicines and Healthcare products Regulatory Agency
Welwyn Garden City, UK

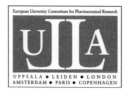

European University Consortium for Pharmaceutical Research

UPPSALA • LEIDEN • LONDON
AMSTERDAM • PARIS • COPENHAGEN

London • Chicago

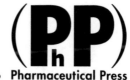

Pharmaceutical Press

Published by the Pharmaceutical Press
An imprint of RPS Publishing

1 Lambeth High Street, London SE1 7JN, UK
100 South Atkinson Road, Suite 200, Grayslake, IL 60030-7820, USA

© Pharmaceutical Press 2007

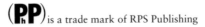 is a trade mark of RPS Publishing

RPS Publishing is the wholly-owned publishing organisation of the
Royal Pharmaceutical Society of Great Britain

First published 2007

Typeset by Type Study, Scarborough, North Yorkshire
Printed in Great Britain by TJ International, Padstow, Cornwall

ISBN 978 0 85369 686 5

A catalogue record for this book is available from the British Library

Contents

ULLA postgraduate pharmacy series

Series Editors-in-Chief

Professor Alexander T Florence and **Professor Anthony C Moffat**, The School of Pharmacy, University of London

The ULLA series is a new and innovative series of introductory textbooks for postgraduate students in the pharmaceutical sciences.

This new series is produced by the ULLA Consortium (European University Consortium for Advanced Pharmaceutical Education and Research). The Consortium is a European academic collaboration in research and teaching of the pharmaceutical sciences that is constantly growing and expanding. The Consortium was founded in 1990 and consists of pharmacy departments from leading universities throughout Europe:

- Faculty of Pharmacy, University of Uppsala, Sweden
- The School of Pharmacy, University of London, UK
- Leiden/Amsterdam Centre for Drug Research, University of Leiden, The Netherlands
- Leiden/Amsterdam Centre for Drug Research, Free University, Amsterdam, The Netherlands
- The Danish University of Pharmaceutical Sciences, Copenhagen, Denmark
- Faculty of Pharmacy, University Paris South, France
- Faculty of Pharmacy, University of Parma, Italy.

The editorial board for the ULLA series consists of several academics from these leading European Institutions who are all experts in their individual field of pharmaceutical science.

The titles in this new groundbreaking series are primarily aimed at European PhD students and will also have global appeal to postgraduate students undertaking masters or diploma courses, undergraduates for specific courses and practising pharmaceutical scientists.

Further information on the Consortium can be found at www.u-l-l-a.org.

Preface

Children form a large percentage of the patient population, but they have been a neglected group where medicines are concerned. It is not that children do not have access to medicines, but that few products have been designed and tested specifically for paediatric use. Children are not simply small adults and, although numerous, are not a homogeneous population. The change in the metabolism and pharmacokinetics of drugs in children is rapid in the first few weeks and months of life and even as the child grows the methodology of calculating doses is not precise.

Because of these factors, markets for children's medicines tend to be small and the range of doses used may be wide for any drug formulation, leading to a lack of attention to paediatric medicines. Because of the paucity of medicines designed and researched specifically for children, the normal regulatory processes for approval of safety and efficacy have been circumvented. Many children are treated with adult medicines used 'off-licence', employing to the full the skill and judgement of physicians and pharmacists to ensure appropriate drug, dose form and dosing regimen. The notion that it is unethical to trial drugs in children holds no force against the ethical issues raised by the use of medicines that have not undergone the same rigorous licensing that adult medicines have to undergo by law.

The situation is changing, and not before time. In the USA incentives are provided to manufacturers through patent extensions for products trialled in children. In the UK, the recent institution and publication of the *BNF for Children* has codified knowledge on the safe use of medicines in children.

This new textbook, not least because it deals with the pharmacokinetics and pharmacodynamics of drugs and formulations in children of different ages, also provides a timely discussion of pharmacogenomics and addresses the real problem of medication errors in paediatric practice, often caused by the need to manipulate adult dose forms to deliver drugs to very young people. There are many challenges in the formulation of established, new and orphan drugs for use in paediatric practice. Some of these are discussed in Chapter 4. This is surely an area for more research in the future. If we can produce nanomedicines we can surely produce delivery systems for the neonate. The text also includes a survey of the regulatory processes for paediatric medicines throughout the world. Without clinical trials in children there can be no comfort in the safety of many therapeutic approaches. Chapter 6 deals not only with the ethics of trials in children but also with trial design in the case of rare diseases, where patient numbers will be limited.

Many of the authors have been or are associated with the Centre for Paediatric Pharmacy Research, the joint venture between the School of Pharmacy, University of London and the Institute of Child Health, University College London. In its short existence this has made a considerable impact in drawing attention to many of the above issues. This book is one of the fruits of this essential collaboration.

Alexander T Florence
Emeritus Dean,
The School of Pharmacy, University of London
October 2006

About the authors

Ian Costello has been a paediatric pharmacist for over 18 years at a number of different hospitals. He was the first Lead Editor of the *BNF for Children* (BNFC) and is now Deputy Chief Pharmacist at St George's Hospital, London. He is an honorary lecturer at the Centre for Paediatric Research and at the School of Pharmacy, University of London and has been the chair of the Neonatal and Paediatric Pharmacists Group for 2005–7.

Paul F Long is a molecular microbiologist whose research sits at the interface of chemistry, biology and clinical pharmaceutics. He has worked in natural product drug discovery in both the health service and pharmaceutical industry, as well as more recently in academia with international collaborations spanning Europe, Japan, the USA and Australia. His interests extend to applying pharmacogenomics to problems in paediatric clinical pharmacy from the use of natural product-derived therapeutics.

Professor Ian K Wong qualified as a pharmacist in 1992. He worked at the former Medicines Control Agency on the Yellow Card system, at the David Lewis Centre for Epilepsy, Northwick Park Hospital and the University of Bradford. In 2002, Professor Wong set up the Centre for Paediatric Pharmacy Research in the School of Pharmacy, University of London, Great Ormond Street Hospital for Children and Institute of Child Health, University of London. His main research interests are paediatric drug safety and health service research. He was awarded a Department of Health Public Health Career Scientist Award in 2002 and Chemists and Druggists Pharmacy Practice Research Medal in 2004 for his research in paediatric medicines.

With a background in pharmaceutical technology and biopharmaceutics, Catherine Tuleu's leading theme of research is on formulation for gastrointestinal drug delivery with emphasis on colonic targeting, where she developed expertise in *in vitro*, and animal and clinical evaluation. Since 2003, she has been leading innovative research in drug delivery for children. Outside the laboratory, she is involved with undergraduate and postgraduate teaching and runs a module on paediatric drug delivery.

Vincent Yeung has recently joined the Medicines and Healthcare products Regulatory Agency (MHRA) as a Good Clinical Practice Inspector. He had been working at Great Ormond Street Hospital for 17 years; he has specialised in clinical trials, research ethics, and metabolic and HIV medicine. He is an honorary lecturer at the Centre for Paediatric Research, University of London. *His views in this book do not represent the view or official position of the MHRA.*

1

Paediatric pharmacokinetics and pharmacodynamics

Ian Costello

Introduction

As knowledge of the physiology of growth and development has increased, it has emerged that the developmental changes that occur throughout a child's life affect the response to drugs and the dose required to achieve a therapeutic effect. The use of equations to estimate children's doses based on those of adults has now been replaced by expressing the dose adjusted for either body weight (mg/kg) or body surface area (mg/m^2) in an attempt to take account of such developmental changes. The more recent integration of developmental pharmacology into paediatric therapeutics has led to a further realisation that such doses are useful to initiate treatment but need to be adjusted for each child, based on developmental differences in pharmacokinetics or pharmacodynamics and response.

Although the most dramatic changes occur in the first 12 months of life, a knowledge of the physiological and developmental changes that occur throughout the child's life and their potential to affect the disposition and action of drugs is essential for safe and effective drug treatment and investigation.

Age ranges and definitions

Perhaps surprisingly, there has been a variation in the definition of the terms 'infant', 'child' and 'adolescent' between texts or studies. To overcome this, the International Commission on Harmonization has defined these terms for regulatory purposes (European Agency for the Evaluation of Medicinal Products, 2000). These definitions and age bands (Table 1.1) broadly represent the ages at which the major changes

Table 1.1 Definitions and age ranges of the paediatric population

Definition	Age range
Preterm newborn infants	< 37 weeks' gestation
Term newborn infants	0–27 days
Infants and toddlers	28 days to 23 months
Children	2–11 years
Adolescents	12–16 or 18 years, depending on region

in physiological, pharmacokinetic and pharmacodynamic parameters occur during development.

Absorption

Oral absorption

Differences

Developmental differences in gastric acid secretion, gastrointestinal motility and drug-metabolising enzymes in the intestinal wall are the main influences on the rate and extent of oral drug absorption. Drugs are chemicals and the chemical environment to which they are exposed will influence their physicochemical properties and therefore their absorption. The majority of drugs are designed to be absorbed from the 'normal' chemical environment of an adult gastrointestinal system.

In term neonates the gastric pH varies between 6 and 8 at birth, dropping to 2–3 within the following few hours. After 24 hours the gastric pH rises again to pH 6–7, gradually falling to reach adult values by 20–30 months (Ritschel and Kearns, 1999). In premature neonates this high gastric pH is prolonged. The physicochemical characteristics of drugs, such as ionisation, will therefore be different in such an environment and may affect the extent of oral absorption when compared with older children or adults. As molecules must be unionised to be absorbed, the extent or rate of absorption of basic drugs may be expected to be increased and those of acidic drugs (phenytoin, phenobarbital) decreased during this period (Morselli *et al.*, 1980). Different oral doses may be required to achieve therapeutic plasma concentrations (e.g. larger doses of phenobarbital on a weight [mg/kg] basis).

The rate at which drugs are absorbed is determined by gastric emptying and intestinal motility. Although the physiology and development of gastrointestinal motility have been studied, there have been few studies of the effects on drug absorption and bioavailability. Generally, the rate at which most drugs are absorbed may be expected to be slower in neonates and young infants up to the age of 4–6 months than in older children (Heimann, 1980) and the time to achieve maximum plasma levels is therefore increased.

Disease states may also influence oral drug absorption. Vomiting or diarrhoea may reduce absorption and result in acutely reduced therapeutic efficacy in chronic diseases such as epilepsy. Gastro-oesophageal reflux disease (GORD) can affect absorption and may require dose alteration as the disease is treated; oral absorption of drugs may be reduced, necessitating higher oral doses initially which may require subsequent reduction once the GORD is controlled.

Another, though less well-characterised, determinant of oral drug absorption is biliary function, which affects the ability to solubilise and absorb lipophilic drugs. Immature transportation and secretion of biliary salts in the neonatal period may affect drug absorption.

Drug absorption and bioavailability are also influenced by intestinal drug-metabolising enzymes and efflux transporters. The developmental changes that occur have not been well studied, although the intestinal mucosal wall activity of cytochrome P450 enzymes may vary with age (Stahlberg et al., 1988; Hesselink et al., 2003).

Variable rates of colonisation of gastrointestinal microflora and beta-glucuronidase activity may also add to the variation and unpredictability of oral drug absorption in neonates and young infants.

Practical implications

Oral absorption of drugs is unpredictable in the neonatal period and for this reason the oral route is not often used to treat acute conditions during this period. Once full feeds have been established oral absorption may be more predictable. Disease states can affect oral absorption in children of all ages and the acute effects should be considered for children with chronic diseases.

Intramuscular absorption

Differences

The rate and extent of absorption of a drug administered intramuscularly depend on blood flow to the muscle. Muscular contractions may also have an influence by affecting drug dispersion.

Reduced skeletal muscle mass, reduced muscle blood flow and

inefficient contractions make intramuscular drug absorption slower and unpredictable in neonates, particularly if premature or paralysed. The physicochemical environment, influenced by acidosis or alkalosis, and muscle physiology may also have an influence in the neonatal period, particularly when preterm. The reduced muscle mass in premature neonates may also predispose to muscle damage if too great a volume of drug is injected.

Absorption of drugs given intramuscularly may be unpredictable if muscle activity is reduced, such as in children who are paralysed or heavily sedated in intensive care, or when blood supply to the muscle is reduced, such as in shock.

Intramuscular injection is generally avoided in children as it is painful and distressing, but it is useful for single injections or to avoid missing doses if the intravenous route is temporarily unavailable.

Practical implications

Consideration should be given to the child's clinical condition and the potential influence on absorption before a drug is administered intramuscularly.

Rectal absorption

Rectal absorption of drugs may be slow and unpredictable in the neonatal period, although it is a useful route when other methods are not available. The relative bioavailability may also be influenced by the rate of hepatic metabolism. The absorption of drugs from the rectum is also influenced by the rate of expulsion. Infants have a greater number of rectal contractions than adults (Di Lorenzo *et al.*, 1995), which may enhance the expulsion of the dose and reduce absorption of drugs such as paracetamol (van Lingen *et al.*, 1999).

Percutaneous absorption

Differences

Differences in the structure, perfusion and hydration of the skin influence percutaneous absorption of drugs. The stratum corneum layer is thinner in preterm neonates and enhanced percutaneous absorption can occur (Rutter, 1987). The greater cutaneous perfusion and epidermal hydration throughout childhood, relative to adults, may also influence percutaneous absorption (Fluhr *et al.*, 2000). The ratio of body surface area to body mass in neonates, infants and young children is far greater than in adults, and therefore the relative systemic exposure of infants and children to drugs applied to the skin may be significantly greater than in adults and can lead to toxicity (Goutieres and Aicardi, 1977; West *et al.*, 1981).

In older children, significant absorption above normal expectations is likely only when large areas of skin are damaged or inflamed. Examples include children with significant burns, psoriasis or eczema.

Enhanced percutaneous absorption may offer a possible route of administration for some drugs, although more research is needed.

Practical implications

When preparations are applied to the skin of infants, particularly preterm neonates, the potential for systemic absorption of excipients as well as any active drug should always be considered.

Renal elimination

Differences

Developmental changes in renal function, particularly glomerular filtration and active tubular secretion, affect the renal excretion of many drugs. In the preterm neonate the kidney is still undergoing development or nephrogenesis. Renal function at birth, and how it develops after birth, are related to the maturity of the developing nephrons.

In neonates over 1.5 kg glomerular filtration rate (GFR) increases dramatically in the first 2 weeks following birth due to adaptive changes in renal blood flow and the recruitment of mature, functioning nephrons. In term neonates the GFR is approximately 2–4 mL/min per 1.73 m^2 at birth and increases rapidly over the following 2–3 weeks (Arant, 1978). Renal tubular secretion increases more slowly but at 8–12 months of age both glomerular and tubular function are close to values seen in adults (Ritschel and Kearns, 1999).

In preterm neonates GFR may be as low as 0.6–0.8 mL/min per 1.73 m^2 and any increase will be determined by the rate of continuing nephrogenesis after birth. Dose intervals of renally excreted drugs must take into account the development and variability of renal function in the neonatal period to avoid potential toxicity and must be individualised to reflect maturational and treatment-associated changes in renal function. Aminoglycosides have been particularly well studied and dose intervals as long as 36–48 hours may be required in preterm neonates to avoid accumulation.

Practical implications

Dose regimens of renally eliminated drugs in neonates are generally based on postconceptional or postmenstrual age as a measure of renal maturation, and postnatal age, to take into account the adaptive changes that occur after birth. However, these should be regarded as initial doses and dose frequency and should be adjusted according to response.

Drug metabolism

Differences

Drugs may be metabolised in the body by enzymes mainly present in the liver. Metabolising enzymes are also present to a lesser extent in the gastrointestinal wall and kidney. These enzymes exist to perform organic functions in the body, but recognise structures present in drug molecules and therefore also transform these structures. It is not surprising that the amount and activity of these enzymes vary with age, maturation, gender and genetic constitution as the body has different organic requirements.

As a consequence, developmental variations in the metabolic fate of drugs can occur and are apparent for many phase I (primarily oxidation, cytochrome P450) and phase II (conjugation) enzymes.

The appearance and activity, or expression, of phase I enzymes changes markedly during development. Changes in the expression of cytochrome P450 (CYP) enzymes occur during fetal development and in the first few hours, weeks and months after birth. For example, the elimination half-life of phenytoin in preterm infants is approximately 75 hours at birth and decreases to 24–48 hours in term infants; the half-life further decreases after birth to approximately 8 hours by 14 days' postnatal age (Loughnan et al., 1977). The elimination half-life of theophylline decreases linearly with postnatal age from 8–18 hours in term infants to 3–4 hours by 48 weeks of life (Nasif et al., 1981). The activity of the enzyme system responsible for the hepatic metabolism of carbamazepine (CYP3A4) is higher in children and a gradual change to adult levels occurs during adolescence (Korinthenberg et al., 1994). The enzymes CYP3A4 and -5 are also present in the gastrointestinal wall and changes in the expression of these enzymes can influence oral drug absorption and bioavailability. Recent studies have shown that puberty, genetic polymorphism and disease states such as cystic fibrosis also influence the expression of CYP enzymes.

Several phase II enzymes may also be expressed as a function of age. Studies of paracetamol (acetaminophen) suggest that sulfation is the major metabolic pathway during the neonatal period and early infancy, changing to glucuronidation over several months (Miller *et al.*, 1976). The increase in morphine clearance due to glucuronidation is related to postconceptional age (Scott *et al.*, 1999).

Practical implications

The expression of metabolising enzymes can affect the therapeutic dose and efficacy of drugs. The rate of metabolism of drugs is often age dependent and may exceed adult values at some stages of development, requiring higher weight-based doses. Initially effective doses in the first few days after birth may require increases in dose or dose frequency to maintain therapeutic efficacy as the child develops and metabolism increases. The metabolites produced may also be different at different stages of life and can influence the potential for toxicity and efficacy.

Distribution

Differences

Changes in body composition that occur during development alter the way that drugs are distributed round the body. The most dramatic changes in body composition occur in the first year of life but changes continue throughout development through puberty and adolescence, particularly the proportion of total body fat.

Neonates and infants have relatively large extracellular fluid and total body water spaces compared with adults, resulting in a larger apparent volume of distribution of drugs that distribute into these spaces (such as aminoglycosides) and lower plasma concentrations for the same weight-based dose. Neonatal adipose tissue also contains a higher proportion of water than that of adults, which may further increase the apparent volume of distribution.

Plasma protein binding is altered in neonates and young infants due to changes in the amount and composition of circulating plasma proteins, such as albumin and α_1-acid glycoprotein. For a given concentration of a drug in the plasma a proportion will be bound to plasma protein and a proportion will be unbound. Only non-protein-bound drug in the plasma is able to distribute to its site of action and is called the free or active fraction. For drugs that are highly protein bound only a small fraction of the concentration measured in the plasma is unbound, and small changes in the binding of the drug can make a large difference to the free drug concentration.

Quantities of albumin and total plasma protein in neonates and young infants are reduced: during the neonatal period fetal albumin is present in plasma and has a reduced binding affinity for some drugs; and endogenous substances such as bilirubin and free fatty acids may displace a drug from its protein-binding site. All these factors may contribute to a higher and variable free fraction of highly protein-bound drugs in neonates and young infants. Lower total plasma concentrations of some drugs may be required to achieve a therapeutic effect. Drugs affected include phenytoin, phenobarbital and furosemide.

As most of the distribution of a drug occurs by passive diffusion along a concentration gradient and subsequent binding of the drug to tissue components, other factors associated with development of disease can influence drug distribution. These include variability in blood flow, organ perfusion, permeability of cell membranes or organs, changes in acid–base balance and cardiac output. The blood–brain barrier may be functionally incomplete in neonates, enabling greater perfusion in the central nervous system. The permeability of organs such as the heart may influence the potential for adverse effects.

Practical implications

The distribution of a drug to its site of action and to other areas of the body affects therapeutic efficacy and adverse effects. Plasma concentrations of drugs may vary considerably in neonates and young infants and distribution, localisation and retention in organs and tissues may be unpredictable. The result may be a different efficacy or adverse effect profile from that expected.

Pharmacodynamics

Although little is known about the effect of development on the interaction between drugs and receptors and the consequences of these interactions (pharmacodynamics), interesting evidence is emerging that age-dependent differences may exist in the interactions of drugs with receptors (warfarin, ciclosporin) or the relationship between plasma concentration and effect (midazolam).

Age-dependent differences in the incidence or severity of adverse effects, such as the increased hepatic toxicity of valproate in infants, may also be due to pharmacodynamic determinants.

Calculating doses in children

Choosing the appropriate dose for a child can present some difficulties. Most doses of drugs have been derived from trials or from clinical experience and are expressed as milligrams per kilogram of body weight (mg/kg). Doses are expressed in formularies in this way for different age ranges of children (e.g. child 2–6 years 10 mg/kg twice daily; child 6–12 years 10 mg/kg three times daily). This assumes that the body weight is appropriate for the child's age. However, this may not be the case due to disease states, prematurity or obesity. Children also grow at different rates. Before a dose is decided upon the appropriateness of the child's weight for age and height should be assessed.

Using body surface area may be the most accurate method for calculating doses, as surface area better reflects changes in cardiac output, fluid requirements, body composition and renal function. However, determining surface area can be time-consuming when prescribing for children and this method of dose calculation is generally reserved for potent drugs where there are small differences between efficacious and toxic doses (e.g. cytotoxic drugs).

Age bands are a practical method for calculating doses of drugs with a wide safety margin in appropriate dose, but the appropriateness of the dose for the individual child, who may be small or large for the age, should also be assessed.

Formulations

Appropriate formulations to enable administration of drugs to children are often not available. Children are often unable to swallow tablets or capsules. Crushing of tablets or manipulation of solid dosage forms into suspensions or powders is often required. Little information may be available on the bioavailability of such formulations (see Chapter 4).

Conclusion: practical applications of developmental changes to treatment

The known variations in pharmacokinetics and the significant gaps in knowledge that exist mean that it is not possible to use simple formulae or allometric scaling to determine the appropriate safe and effective dose for a child from a known adult dose.

Developmental changes produce differences in the absorption, metabolism and excretion of drugs. These age-related changes in pharmacokinetics have been used as determinants in the development of age-specific dose recommendations.

Most doses for children are based on weight as it is an easily measurable parameter, although body surface area may reflect physiological differences more accurately.

Age-related changes in pharmacokinetics can result in a variable and unpredictable response to drugs, particularly in preterm neonates, term neonates and young infants. Dose recommendations should generally be regarded as a good starting point. Knowledge of the influence of development on the factors that may affect the response to drugs is essential in adjusting treatment to maximise efficacy and minimise adverse effects.

References

Arant B S (1978). Developmental patterns of renal functional maturation compared in the human neonate. *J Pediatr* 92: 705–712.

Di Lorenzo C, Flores C F, Hyman P E (1995). Age related changes in colon motility. *J Pediatr* 127: 593–596.

European Agency for the Evaluation of Medicinal Products (2000). ICH Topic E11 Note for guidance on clinical investigation of medicinal products in the paediatric population (CPMP/ICH/2711/99). London: EMEA.

Fluhr J W, Pfisterer S, Gloor M (2000). Direct comparison of skin physiology in children and adults with bioengineering methods. *Paediatr Dermatol* 17: 436–439.

Goutieres F, Aicardi J (1977). Accidental percutaneous hexachlorophane intoxication in children. *BMJ* ii: 663–665.

Heimann G (1980). Enteral absorption and bioavailability in children in relation to age. *Eur J Clin Pharmacol* 18: 43–50.

Hesselink D A, van Schaik R H, van der Heiden I P, *et al.* (2003). Genetic polymorphisms of the CYP3A4, CYP3A5, and MDR-1 genes and pharmacokinetics of the calcineurin inhibitors cyclosporine and tacrolimus. *Clin Pharmacol Ther* 74: 245–254.

Korinthenberg R, Haug C, Hannak D (1994). The metabolization of carbamazepine to CBZ-10,11-epoxide in children from the newborn age to adolescence. *Neuropediatrics* 25: 214–216.

Loughnan P, Greenwald A, Purton W W, *et al.* (1977). Pharmacokinetic observations of phenytoin disposition in the newborn and young infant. *Arch Dis Child* 52: 302–309.

Miller R P, Roberts R J, Fischer L J (1976). Acetaminophen elimination kinetics in neonates, children and adults. *Clin Pharmacol Ther* 19: 284–294.

Morselli P L, Franco-Morselli R, Bossi L (1980). Clinical pharmacokinetics in newborns and infants, age related differences and therapeutic implications. *Clin Pharmacokinet* 5: 485–527.

Nasif E G, Weinberger M M, Shannon D, *et al.* (1981). Theophylline disposition in infancy. *J Pediatr* 98: 158–161.

Ritschel W A, Kearns G L (1999). Paediatric pharmacokinetics. In: *Handbook of Basic Pharmacokinetics*, 5th edn. Washington DC: American Pharmaceutical Association, 304–321.

Rutter N (1987). Percutaneous drug absorption in the newborn: hazards and uses. *Clin Perinatol* 14: 911–930.

Scott C S, Riggs K W, Ling E W, *et al.* (1999). Morphine pharmacokinetics and pain assessment in premature newborns. *J Pediatr* 135: 423–429.

Stahlberg M R, Hietanen E, Maki M (1988). Mucosal biotransformation rates in the small intestine of children. *Gut* 29: 1058–1063.

van Lingen R A, Deinum J T, Quak J M, *et al.* (1999). Pharmacokinetics and metabolism of rectally administered paracetamol in preterm neonates. *Arch Dis Child Fetal Neonatal Ed* 80: F59–F63.

West D P, Worobec S, Solomon L M (1981). Pharmacology and toxicology of infant skin. *J Invest Dermatol* 76: 147–150.

2

Pharmacogenomic considerations in paediatric drug handling

Paul F Long

Pharmacogenomics in a paediatric setting – some history and definitions

It is now over 50 years since Watson and Crick described the structure of DNA, postulating a copying mechanism that provides a chemical basis for genetic transmission and a scientific basis for mendelian inheritance of traits. In the intervening five decades we have gone from sequencing relatively short pieces of DNA to having the enabling technologies to sequence entire genomes, culminating in 2001 with completion of the Human Genome Project (Lander *et al.*, 2001; Venter *et al.*, 2001). Deciphering the human genome has led to an explosion in genetic tools to diagnose, manage and treat diseases. Physicians have long been aware of subtle differences in our inter-individual response to medication. What is still poorly understood is how the genes controlling our growth and development, from conception to birth and on through to adulthood, might also interact with gene networks that influence our response to particular medicines – this is a paediatric model exemplifying the science of pharmacogenomics. Being able to predict atypical drug responses will allow the dose of medicines for children to be individually tailored and adapted to avoid toxicity and maximise clinical efficacy; however, the consequences of drug action might well be different depending on the stage of development.

DNA is a linear polymer consisting of a deoxyribose phosphate backbone to which monomeric subunits comprising the bases adenine, thymine, cytosine and guanine are attached. The unit consisting of sugar, phosphate and base is referred to as a nucleotide. The complete haploid human genome has around 3.2 billion of these nucleotides which can be arranged in any order, but a key feature is the consistent Chargaff pairings of A–T, G–C. The chain forms a double helix and the integrity of this helix is maintained by internal hydrogen bonding of the bases and between adjacent loops of the helix. The nucleotides are distributed across 22 autosomes and 1 sex chromosome, either X or Y. Somatic cells are diploid, containing maternal and paternal copies of each chromosome, giving a total of 46 in all. Each gene is, therefore, duplicated at any given locus and can be described as dominant, co-dominant or recessive. A sequence of nucleotides that is necessary for the synthesis of a functional polypeptide is the simplest definition of a gene. The human genome consists of around 45 000 genes. Each gene is composed of groups of nucleotides called exons, which carry the genetic code, separated by alternating groups of nucleotides, the non-coding introns, which are essential for regulating transcription and translation of the genetic code.

Proteins make up essential structural constituents of cells and mediate biochemical reactions as either regulatory molecules or enzyme catalysts. Many proteins are important in drug pharmacokinetics and pharmacodynamics, which explains why variability in response to therapeutic interventions can have an inherited basis. In addition to the genes found within the nucleus of each reproductive and somatic cell, genes are also located in the maternally inherited mitochondria. The term 'genomics' not only was coined to describe the effects of single genes themselves, but also in recent years has been expanded to include the biological processes controlling the function of gene networks, including environment–gene interactions (Evans and Relling, 1999).

There are approximately three million differences between the DNA sequences of any two copies of the human genome. In other words, all individuals are genetically 99.9% similar, so only 0.1% of the genome is responsible for all the genetic diversity between men and women, or between individuals from different ethnic and racial groupings. This variation is most often the result of a single-point mutation in base pairing that results in the substitution of a nucleotide and is called a single nucleotide polymorphism (SNP). There are estimated to be at least 1.4 million different SNPs that are physically distributed throughout the entire human genome. The majority of SNPs have no deleterious effects; however, if the SNP occurs in a coding region of the genome, and approximately 60 000 do, a protein can be synthesised with an abnormal phenotype if a crucial change in an amino acid occurs. Multiple SNPs in the same region of the genome that are also inherited together more strongly influence phenotype than individual SNPs; these are referred to as an individual's haplotype (Sachidanandam *et al.*, 2001).

Clinical observations of inherited differences in drug effects have been recognised for many years, a classic example being haemolysis among African–American soldiers in the US army taking the anti-malarial primaquine during World War II. Another notable milestone in studying genetic variation in drug metabolism came in 1960 from observations that inherited deficiencies in serum cholinesterase led to differing susceptibility to muscle relaxants and that individuals could be described as either 'slow' or 'rapid' drug metabolisers. This led to the realisation that administering a standard dose of medicine to these 'slow' metabolisers, or to individuals with genetic deficiencies in enzymes responsible for drug deposition, could lead to adverse or even fatal drug reactions. It is estimated that over 100 000 deaths in the USA can be attributed annually to these iatrogenic affects. Conversely, individuals with an inherited 'rapid' metabolism are at risk as non-responders to treatment failure; again this could prove fatal when treating certain life-threatening conditions, particularly cancer or HIV infection.

The relevance to clinical outcome of a genetic polymorphism in drug metabolism enzymes can differ, based on dosing of the treatment regimen prescribed. When dosing is comparatively modest, then inheriting an enzyme deficiency can increase exposure to the medication without the risk of inducing an adverse effect, thereby increasing efficacy over a longer treatment period. Conversely, when drugs are dosed at levels near to toxic, then inheritance of an enzyme deficiency could be detrimental, leading to an overdose because the medication cannot be adequately cleared.

Built on the pioneering work of Archibald Garrod in the early part of the twentieth century studying the 'inborn errors of metabolism', Frederick Vogel coined the term 'pharmacogenetics' in 1959 to explain inter-individual and inter-racial differences in drug metabolism. This term has largely been superseded today by 'pharmacogenomics' to incorporate a much wider understanding of genetic differences in all aspects of drug disposition, including genetic variation in genes encoding drug transporters that influence drug absorption, distribution and excretion, and also pharmacodynamic characteristics or protein drug targets (Kalow, 2005). In reality the two terms are commonly interchangeable; however, pharmacogenomics is more attractive when considered in a paediatric setting because this definition captures both the effects of developmental genes and the genes involved in drug deposition, and the action on the overall process of drug response.

Development is a continuum, from conception, fetal maturation, neonatal growth through to childhood and adolescence. The patterns of gene expression will change with age and so the nature of gene interactions that could contribute to drug response might be relevant only at specific and discernible time points that can be expected to change as a child grows. Observable consequences of drug exposure during development could be immediate, such as *in utero* death or malformation. Alternatively, these consequences may not be discernible until later life, for example, effects on cognitive function or behaviour.

Paediatric pharmacogenomics in drug metabolism and drug response

The human genome encodes some 30 families of drug-metabolising enzymes, most of which have genetic variants causing functional changes in these enzymes, altering drug metabolism (Ingelman-Sundberg and Rodriguez-Antona, 2005). As is typical for many gene polymorphisms, there are important racial and ethnic differences in the frequencies of gene mutations in different human populations. The cytochrome P450 (CYP) enzymes represent the largest of these families, with genetic polymorphism in debrisoquin hydroxylase (*CYP2D6*), the first and probably best characterised. A large number of *CYP2D6* SNPs have been documented, and concordance between genotype and phenotype well established for many drug substrates particularly relevant to paediatric drug handling. For example, deficiency in CYP2D6 can result in diminished analgesic effects since CYP2D6 is required for activation of codeine, the most common form of pain relief given in postoperative paediatric settings. Likewise, deficiency in CYP2D6 can also lead to exaggerated drug effects in children when this CYP is the major metabolising enzyme of, for example, tricyclic antidepressants. Conversely, inheritance of an 'ultra-rapid metaboliser' phenotype has also been linked to treatment failure in children and adolescents prescribed the selective serotonin reuptake inhibitor (SSRI) group of antidepressant and antipsychotic drugs.

Exposure of an unborn fetus to drugs during pregnancy as a consequence of either maternal drug therapy or substance abuse can be associated with an increased risk of fetal malformation, growth retardation or even *in utero* death. The ability to identify individuals at risk of these undesirable effects would be a significant advantage, particularly when exposure to drugs cannot be avoided. Consequently, assessing protective barriers at the fetal–maternal interface against embryotoxic or teratogenic drugs is of considerable interest.

Maintaining the integrity of the conceptus as it grows and develops involves the placenta and both maternal and fetal drug biotransformation and transporter systems. The human placenta is able to metabolise some drugs and several enzyme and transporter systems have been identified including CYP enzymes. There is evidence for constitutive CYP activity not found in adults (CYP3A7 and CYP1A1) and other CYPs that are inducible in response to maternal recreational drug abuse (CYP2E1). Little is known about placental allelic variation in CYP enzymes or the effect that these variations have on enzyme activity.

Genetic polymorphism of thiopurine methyltransferase (TPMT) is a classic example of clinical pharmacogenomics, with about 90% of individuals expressing a highly active enzyme phenotype, 10% an enzyme with immediate activity and 0.3% with low or undetectable levels of enzyme activity. Thiopurine agents such as azathioprine, mercaptopurine and thioguanine are used in the treatment of a range of conditions, principally leukaemia. As prodrugs, these agents are activated to form thioguanine nucleotides that are incorporated into DNA to exert their cytotoxic effects. The drugs can be inactivated via either oxidation by xanthine oxidase or S-methylation by TPMT. In haematopoietic tissues, xanthine oxidase is negligible, leaving TPMT as the only inactivation pathway. Individuals, especially children, with low or undetectable enzyme activity are at high risk of severe and often fatal bone marrow suppression.

The molecular basis for polymorphic TPMT activity has been located to eight alleles, with three alleles designated *TPMT*2*, *TPMT*3A* and *TPMT*3C* accounting for about 95% of all intermediate or low enzyme activity phenotypes. When an individual is homozygous for any variant alleles, then the individual is TPMT deficient. When an individual is heterozygous, inheriting one wild-type allele and any one of the variant alleles, then the individual will express an enzyme with intermediate activity. So patients with a homozygous mutant or heterozygous genotype are at very high risk of developing severe haematopoietic toxicity, if treated with conventional doses of thiopurines.

A study of mercaptopurine use in childhood leukaemia found that TPMT-deficient patients failed to tolerate full doses of mercaptopurine in 76% of scheduled weeks of treatment, whereas heterozygous and homozygous wild-type patients failed to tolerate full doses for 16% and 2% of treatment weeks respectively. Although the influence of TPMT genotype on bone marrow suppression is most dramatic for homozygous mutant patients, the failure rate among heterozygotes at 16% is also of clinical relevance, representing approximately 10% of children treated with mercaptopurine. Homozygous mutant or compound heterozygote children with a 'low methylator' status may tolerate standard doses, but are at significantly greater risk of toxicity, often necessitating a lower dose of these drugs. TPMT genotyping is the first Clinical Laboratory Improvement Amendments (CLIA)-certified pharmacogenomic test for individualising drug treatment based on a genotype.

Transport proteins such as the ATP-binding cassette (ABC) family of membrane transporters play an important part in overcoming biological barriers, influencing the absorption of many drugs. P-glycoprotein (PGP) is a member of this family and is involved in the energy-dependent efflux of drugs and their metabolites into urine, bile, the intestinal lumen and the placenta. Expression of the PGP gene (*ABCB1*, also called *MDR1*) differs markedly among individuals. Recently, a synonymous SNP in exon 26 (3435C>T), was reported to be associated with duodenal PGP protein expression; patients homozygous for the T allele had more than twofold lower duodenal PGP expression than patients with CC genotypes. In a study investigating the pharmacokinetics of the antiretrovirals nelfinavir and efavirenz, which included a paediatric cohort, the *ABCB1* 3435C>T polymorphism was found to be associated with significant differences in recovery of CD4 count. Of all variables evaluated, only *ABCB1* genotype and baseline HIV RNA copy number were significant predictors of this CD4 recovery.

Personalised treatment is a pharmacogenomic goal. This study is the first evidence that a host genetic marker can predict immune recovery after initiation of antiretroviral treatment, suggesting a potential strategy to individualise HIV therapy.

Pharmacogenomics and new paediatric drug targets

In few other therapeutic areas are the concepts of pharmacogenomics better illustrated and the promise more apparent than in the treatment of children (Stephenson, 2005). Issues of adverse drug reactions and non-responsiveness due to poor formulation and dosing are among the most challenging clinical problems in paediatric pharmacy today. Age-related differences in anatomy and physiology readily distinguish children from adults; dosing guidelines developed through clinical trials in adults are, therefore, seldom adequate in a paediatric setting since children tend to eliminate drugs much faster on a milligram per kilogram basis than adults.

There is mounting evidence for a higher incidence of adverse reactions in children compared with adults. Frequently quoted is 'gray baby syndrome' in newborns treated with chloramphenicol due to poor age-dependent expression of the metabolising enzyme glucuronosyl transferase. Unfortunately, drug metabolism is seldom delineated to a single enzyme; more often, either multiple pathways can lead to many metabolites (for example, valproic acid used in the treatment of childhood seizures) or a single metabolite may be formed through a multi-enzyme pathway, with the genes encoding each enzyme disposed to allelic variation (for example, metabolism of 6-mercaptopurine used in the treatment of childhood leukaemia).

Ontogeny of drug metabolism and developmental changes in drug-metabolising phenotypes across the paediatric continuum may hold the key to explaining drug-induced adverse effects; this has important implications for optimising paediatric drug dosing.

Successful implementation of pharmacogenomic strategies also involves an appreciation of pharmacodynamic processes. The aetiology of many diseases affecting children (asthma, autism, attention deficit hyperactivity disorder, epilepsy, certain cancers, Kawasaki's disease) are poorly understood, or have no close correlates in adults, limiting both treatment paradigms and target identification. Furthermore, phenotypic changes in the drug target across the paediatric continuum will influence the relative success of any pharmacotherapy rationale. Receptor polymorphism and response to anti-asthma therapy is a well-cited example.

Cysteinyl leukotrienes are potent bronchoconstrictors implicated in the pathogenesis of asthma. Thus, targeted disruption of the leukotriene pathway is a useful anti-asthmatic treatment, especially in adults. However, not all children with asthma experience clinical improvement from this therapeutic intervention, suggesting that it is the relative level of leukotriene production rather than total antagonism of drug target that influences clinical outcome. The enzyme 5-lipoxygenase is the target for the drug ABT-761. Allelic variation in the promoter region of the gene encoding this enzyme (*ALOX5*) has been associated with clinical response to ABT-761. Individuals with asthma who are homozygous recessive, possessing mutant *ALOX5* alleles, have lower enzyme activity and, therefore, release less leukotriene from their leukocytes. These patients are less responsive to ABT-761 than heterozygotes and those carrying a mutation transversion who produce a relatively greater amount of leukotriene. Disease management in childhood asthma and, presumably, other high-incident paediatric disorders uncommon in adults is related to allelic variation and ontogeny in the receptor.

Pharmacogenomics in paediatric pharmacy practice

Pharmacogenomics offers pharmacists an innovative opportunity to create a new dimension to their practice by accessing genetic services, and expanding current primary delivery in healthcare promotion and patient management (Vizirianakis, 2002; Brock *et al.*, 2003). There is clearly great potential for pharmacogenomics to yield new molecular diagnostics that could become routine tests by which pharmacists select drugs and doses for individual patients. Easy-to-use gene chip technology opens up the possibility of risk assessment, even in community-based settings, to screen individuals with poor metabolising phenotypes, developing personalised treatment plans so that the right patient receives the right drug at the right time. It is already possible at a reasonable cost quickly to test for polymorphisms in CYP genes, which encode for enzymes that play a major role in the way that an individual metabolises drugs.

The ability to distinguish between fast and slow metabolisers would allow prescription and dispensing of appropriate drug doses and the monitoring of an individual's response to treatment simultaneously. Haplotype profiling could become an integral part of a person's medical records, changing the practice of pharmacy so that individualised drug therapy becomes the norm. Although this information offers the potential to design appropriate prevention and intervention priorities, pharmacists must consider and become knowledgeable about their attendant ethical, legal and social responsibilities in handling genetic information. The scope and standards delineating the roles and responsibilities of pharmacists in providing genetic healthcare have yet to be defined, but supporting patient and family empowerment, partnering them to meaningful health decisions and becoming fluent in the management of genetic health information, are just a few of the emerging roles that pharmacogenomics could make a reality for tomorrow's pharmacy graduates.

References

Brock T P, Valgus J M, Smith S R, *et al.* (2003). Pharmacogenomics: implications and considerations for pharmacists. *Pharmacogenomics* 4: 321–330.

Evans W E, Relling M V (1999). Pharmacogenomics: translating functional genomics into rational therapeutics. *Science* 286: 487–491.

Ingelman-Sundberg M, Rodriguez-Antona C (2005). Pharmacogenetics of drug-metabolizing enzymes: implications for a safer and more effective drug therapy. *Phil Trans R Soc Lond B Biol Sci* 360: 1563–1570.

Kalow W (2005). Pharmacogenomics: historical perspective and current status. *Methods Mol Biol.* 311: 3–15.

Lander E S, Linton L M, Birren B, *et al.* (2001). Initial sequencing and analysis of the human genome. *Nature* 409: 860–921.

Sachidanandam R, Weissman D, Schmidt S C, *et al.* (2001). A map of human genome variation containing 1.42 million single nucleotide polymorphisms. *Nature* 409: 928–933.

Stephenson T (2005). How children's responses to drugs differ from adults. *Br J Clin Pharmacol* 59: 670–673.

Venter J C, Adams M D, Myers E W, *et al.* (2001). The sequence of the human genome. *Science* 291: 1304–1351.

Vizirianakis I S (2002). Pharmaceutical education in the wake of genomic technologies for drug development and personalized medicine. *Eur J Pharm Sci* 15: 243–250.

3

Medication errors in children

Ian K Wong

Introduction

Miss Hartigan, a mother of a 9-week-old baby, checked the label on her son's repeat prescription and realised that each pill contained 25 mg instead of 2 mg of captopril. The hospital that had prescribed the drug following surgery confirmed the mistake. She was initially shocked but relieved. Miss Hartigan said 'I understand people do make mistakes but then it happened a second time. I was really upset and angry that something so serious could have happened and was happening again' (BBC News, 2004). Thankfully, Miss Hartigan's experience is not frequent; however, many cases of tenfold medication errors in children have been reported in the literature and many have tragic outcomes. In this chapter you will be introduced to the definition, epidemiology, nature and prevention of medication errors in children.

Definitions of medication error

'Medical error' is an umbrella term given to all errors that occur within the healthcare system, including mishandled surgery, diagnostic errors, equipment failures and medication errors. As medicines are the most common interventions in the healthcare system, medication errors are probably one of the most common types of medical error. Research suggests that approximately 7000 patients a year are killed by medication errors in the USA (Kohn *et al.*, 1999), and in British hospitals the incidence and consequences appear to be similar (Cowley *et al.*, 2001; Dean *et al.*, 2002).

Prescribing, dispensing and administration of medicines for children pose a unique set of risks, predominantly because of the wide variation in body mass, which requires doses to be calculated individually based on patient age, weight or body surface area, and their clinical condition. This increases the likelihood of errors, and tenfold errors, as shown in Miss Hartigan's case, are not rare (Wong *et al.*, 2004). In addition, dosage formulations are often extemporaneously compounded to meet the need for small doses in these patients, and there is a lack of information on paediatric doses and indications. As a result, clinical decision-making is particularly difficult in young children.

In order to study and understand medication errors in children, it is important to define what a paediatric medication error is. Ghaleb and Wong (2006) reviewed various definitions and, to their surprise, found that many research reports did not include any definition. Variations in the definitions limit comparison between studies, as do the methods used. In 2005 Ghaleb and colleagues used the Delphi technique to define prescribing errors in children: 'A clinically meaningful prescribing error occurs when, as a result of a prescribing decision or prescription writing process, there is an unintentional significant: (1) reduction in the probability of treatment being timely and effective or (2) increase in the risk of harm when compared with generally accepted practice'.

Process-based methods for measuring medication errors

Three methods for measuring medication errors have been used in most medication error research: spontaneous reporting, chart review and observation (Wong *et al.*, 2004).

Spontaneous reporting system

The spontaneous reporting system is very similar to the adverse drug reaction reporting system and requires a person who witnesses, commits or discovers an error or near-miss to report it to a central data collection department or organisation such as the UK National Patient Safety Agency. Similar to the adverse drug reaction reporting system, one of the major problems with the spontaneous reporting system is under-estimation due to inability to recognise errors and under-reporting.

Chart review

Chart review involves researchers reviewing prescriptions, prescribing charts or computer-prescribing records to identify medication errors. It is widely used for detecting prescribing errors; however, it relies on the clinical skills of researchers to detect the error, and inter-observer difference (inter-rater reliability) can be problematic when different observers are involved in observation. Chart review is relatively in-effective in detecting administration errors because charts do not usually record the process of drug preparation and administration (see next section for comparison).

Observation

Observation is the most labour-intensive method of measuring medi-cation errors. It involves researchers observing health professionals while they are preparing and administering medications to patients. The researcher records details of all doses administered, and compares this information with the doses prescribed. A major concern with this method is the potential effect on the nurses being observed: they may modify their practice during the observations. Therefore, many obser-vational studies involved the use of disguised techniques where nurses were aware of the observation but unaware of its true purpose (Bruce and Wong, 2001).

Outcome-based method

The chart review and observation are process-based methods for detect-ing errors. Most of these 'process errors', however, do not cause harm, so these methods are not cost-effective for the study of the harmful outcomes of medication errors.

The analysis of harmful spontaneous medication error reports is a popular and cost-effective method for identifying harmful medication errors in order to propose an error reduction strategy. Cousins *et al.* (2002) conducted an analysis of reviewed press reports over an 8-year period. This is a very cost-effective approach to identifying serious and harmful medication errors, but it is unable to provide information on epidemiology.

Incidence of paediatric medication errors

Ghaleb and Wong (2006) reviewed the medication errors published between 1995 and 2004. The results are shown in Tables 3.1–3.3.

The variation in the error rates was probably due to the differences in the definitions of medication errors, the methodologies used and the settings. For example, the error rate in a neonatal intensive care unit is much higher than that in a general paediatric ward. Furthermore, the systems of prescribing, dispensing and drug administration vary

Table 3.1 Studies that used spontaneous reporting as method of detecting medication errors of all types in paediatrics

Reference	Time frame	Setting	Study design	No. of reports/Reporting rate
Paton and Wallace, 1997 (UK)	2 years (April 1994–June 1996)	Paediatric hospital	Analysis of routinely collected medication error reports	Number of reports 92. No reporting rate given
Wilson et al., 1998 (UK)	2 years	Teaching hospital (1 PCW and 1 PCICU)	Analysis of routinely reported medication errors by doctors, nurses and pharmacists. ME reports analysed by committee, who met at 3-monthly intervals to analyse reports. Errors categorised into: AE, SE and PE, serious or not, and outcome	Number of reports 441. Reporting rate 17.2 per 100 admissions
Selbst et al., 1999 (US)	5 years (1991–1996)	Paediatric hospital – emergency department	Review of all ED incident reports to identify errors. Then conducted chart review of all medication and intravenous fluid errors	Number of reports 33. No reporting rate given
Ross et al., 2000 (UK)	5 years (April 1994–March 1999)	Paediatric hospital and NICU in general hospital	Retrospective review of routinely reported medication error reports. Reporting is mandatory in hospital for all staff	Number of reports 195. Reporting rate 0.15 per 100 admissions

AE, administration error; ED, emergency department; ME, medication error; NICU, neonatal intensive care unit; PCICU, paediatric cardiac intensive care unit; PICU, paediatric intensive care unit; PE, prescribing error; PCW, paediatric cardiac ward; DE, dispensing error.

Table 3.2 Studies that used medication order/chart review as a method to detect medication errors of all types in paediatrics

Reference	Time frame	Settings	Study design	Errant medication orders/Error rate
Marino et al., 2000 (USA)	Two phases in summer 1995. Phase 1: 14 days; phase 2: 5 days	Large metropolitan paediatric teaching hospital. Phase 1: 2 units (ICU and medical surgical unit). Phase 2: 3 units (ICU, medical and surgical units)	Prospective study Following medication order written from prescribing through administration. Also review of medical record, pharmacy's clinical interventions and quality control log, and incident reports. Also review of medication administration record Sample = 3312 medication orders	784 errors identified Error rate 24/100 orders Administration error 0.15% doses administered
Kaushal et al., 2001 (USA)[a]	6 weeks (April and May 1999)	All wards in a paediatric teaching hospital and all paediatric wards in a general teaching hospital	Prospective study Identified incidents from reports, medication order sheets and medication administration records and chart reviews Sample = 10 778 medication orders	Errant medication orders 616 orders Error rate 5.7/100 orders
Kozer et al., 2002 (Canada)	12 randomly selected days from summer of 2000	Paediatric hospital – emergency department	Retrospective study Chart review of patients treated in emergency department Sample 1532 charts = no. of patients No. of medication orders = 1678	26.3% of charts contain potential errors 10% of patients subjected to medication errors (10.1% with prescription errors, 3.9% with drug administration errors)
Fontan et al., 2003 (France)	8 weeks	Paediatric hospital	Prospective study Prescription and administration documents were analysed daily and medical record analysis was used to compare the prescription with administration report Sample = 49 patients Prescriptions = 511 Prescribed drugs = 4532	Prescription error rate 20.7% (1.9 errors per patient per day) Administration error rate 23.5%
Cimino et al., 2004 (USA)	2 weeks pre-intervention; 3 month site-specific error reduction interventions; 2 weeks post-intervention	Paediatric hospitals – 9 PICUs	Prospective study Three levels of surveillance used: (1) pharmacy order review for errors and computer order entry step; (2) PICU nurse order transcription and review for errors step; (3) an oversight team check Sample = 12 026 medication orders	Error rate 0.22 per order

[a] This study used combination of methods including review of incident reports.
ICU, intensive care unit; PICU, paediatric intensive care unit.

Table 3.3 Studies that involve observation methods to detect drug administration errors in paediatrics

Reference	Duration of study	Hospital–clinical area	Sample size	Sampling methods	Error rate (excluding wrong time error)
Nixon and Dhillon, 1996 (UK)[a]	2 weeks	General hospital – two paediatric wards (one medical and one surgical)	487 and 425 administration observed for medical and surgical wards respectively. No. of patients not mentioned	Observation from 8am to 8pm, Monday to Saturday	Administration errors 5.6% and 4.5% for respective wards
Schneider et al., 1998 (Switzerland)	10 weeks	Teaching hospital – PICU	20 observation periods (275 drug administrations observed) involving 12 patients	Twice a week observations from 8.30am to 1.30pm	18.2% of administrations
Herout and Erstad, 2004 (USA)	1 month	Tertiary care teaching hospital – SICU	206 infusions involving 71 patients	Observations recorded on a daily basis	105.9 per 1000 patient-days

PICU, paediatric intensive care unit; SICU, surgical intensive care unit.
[a]Prescribing errors were also studied; these were collected and recorded by the pharmacist while monitoring the patients' drug therapy. Prescribing error rate reported was 5.3% or 41 errors/100 beds per week.

significantly between different countries, hence the frequency and causes of error in each country are likely to be different.

Ghaleb and Wong's review (2006) demonstrates that the spontaneous reporting systems tend to yield a lower rate of paediatric medication errors than the other methods. This is due to underestimation and under-reporting. In contrast, observation methods tend to find higher incidences than the other two methods. These published reports confirm that paediatric medication errors are at least as common as errors in adults. A study by Kaushal and colleagues (2001) has shown that potential adverse drug events may be three times more common in children than in adults.

Consequences of errors

The majority of paediatric medications do not result in harm. Blum and co-workers (1988) reported that only 0.2% of the errors could be classified as potentially lethal, whereas Folli *et al.* (1987) reported 5.6% as potentially lethal. Interestingly, no actual harm to children was reported in most of the epidemiological studies. This might be because the errors were identified and rectified before any harm resulted, but it could be due to publication bias – some healthcare providers may be reluctant to publish studies reporting patients with serious harm.

Cousins *et al.* (2002) conducted an analysis of press reports highlighting the outcomes of 24 cases of paediatric medication errors (Table 3.4). Most of the cases reported resulted in fatal consequences, hence making the news headlines.

Types of error

The review by Wong and colleagues concluded that the most common type of paediatric medication errors are dosing errors, especially tenfold errors (Wong *et al.*, 2004). Other paediatric medication errors have been reported in the literature, including:

- Wrong drug
- Wrong route of administration
- Wrong transcription or documentation
- Incorrect or missing date
- Wrong frequency of administration
- Missed dose
- Wrong patient

Table 3.4 Case reports of medication errors in children

Patient involved	Type of error	Description of the error involved	Outcome	Steps taken to prevent future error
1-day-old premature neonate	Incorrect dose – decimal point	Given morphine 15 mg instead of 0.15 mg	Death	Not mentioned
1-day-old baby	Incorrect dose – decimal point	Given 320 mg of i.v. digoxin instead of 32 mg	Death	Not mentioned
Neonate	Incorrect dose – decimal point	Given diamorphine 10 times the dose	Death	Not mentioned
5-year-old girl	Incorrect dose – decimal point	Given tacrolimus 10 times the dose required	Death	Not mentioned
13 year old	Incorrect dose – decimal point and route	Adrenaline 10 times the dose and i.v. instead of i.m.	Allergic reaction (rash and wheezy)	Not mentioned
17 year old	Incorrect dose	i.v. fluids 10 times the dose	Death	Not mentioned
5 year old	Incorrect dose	Anaesthetic, atropine and adrenaline – wrong dose	Heart attack	Not mentioned
9 year old	Incorrect dose	Diamorphine 6 times the dose	Death	Not mentioned
9 year old	Incorrect dose	Oral steroid high dose	Died from chickenpox	Not mentioned
4 year old	Incorrect dose	Growth hormone test overdose	Death	Not mentioned
3-day-old triplet	Incorrect dose	Phenytoin i.v. overdose	Death	Not mentioned
17-month-old infant	Incorrect dose and route	Benzylpenicillin 300 times overdose and injected into spine	Death	Not mentioned
3-month-old baby	Incorrect dose and administration system	Sodium nitroprusside 4 times correct dose and given in the wrong administration system	Death	Not mentioned

Table 3.4 Continued

Patient involved	Type of error	Description of the error involved	Outcome	Steps taken to prevent future error
10 year old	Incorrect drug	Anaesthetic in dental surgery	Death	Not mentioned
14 year old	Incorrect drug	Nitrous oxide/oxygen. The two cylinders had been wrongly connected	Death	Not mentioned
Preterm neonate	Incorrect drug (dialysis fluid)	Dialysis fluid incorrect to the one prescribed	Death	Not mentioned
7 year old	Incorrect drug	Different anaesthetic given to the one prescribed	Death	Not mentioned
12 year old	Incorrect route (intrathecal)	Vincristine given intrathecally instead of i.v.	Death	Not mentioned
4 day old	Incorrect strength	Double-strength chloroform:water concentrate used	Death	Not mentioned
3-day-old preterm	Incorrect rate	i.v. dextrose, infusion rate not controlled	Death	Not mentioned
1 month old	Incorrect rate	Dobutamine, infusion given too rapidly	Death	Not mentioned
11 month old	Incorrect container	Antidepressants from father's medicine not put in childproof container	Death	Not mentioned
Preterm baby	Omitted in error	Potassium chloride was omitted and not put in dialysis fluid	Death	Not mentioned
5 year old	Anaesthesia	Anaesthetic (given general anaesthesia for tooth extraction)	Death	Not mentioned

From Cousins *et al.* (2002).

- Drugs given to patients with known allergies
- Drug interaction
- Intravenous incompatibility
- Omission errors
- Wrong rate of intravenous drug administration.

Methods to identify root causes of medication errors

Although it is important to identify errors, it is far more important to identify the root cause of errors so that changes can be implemented to make the system 'safer'. In the UK, 'clinical governance' requires all healthcare organisations within the National Health Service (NHS) to have a risk management strategy and the National Patient Safety Agency (NPSA) recommends using the human error theory or root cause analysis to achieve safer practice (Gothard *et al.*, 2004). In the USA the Joint Commission on Accreditation of Healthcare Organizations (JCAHO) requires that all healthcare organisations that seek their accreditation perform 'a proactive risk assessment method' annually on any high-risk area and further recommends the use of either healthcare failure mode and effect analysis or root cause analysis (DeRosier *et al.*, 2002).

According to the JCAHO medication error is one of the most important patient safety risk factors. The medical literature describes different models of risk assessment that can be used to identify the causes of medication errors. This is important because without such knowledge no actions would be effective, and furthermore identifying the wrong cause would result in an inappropriate or suboptimal action plan (Weinberg, 2001).

The root cause analysis model

This model originated from the close call reporting system of the National Aeronautics and Space Administration (NASA), which looked at failure in systems and processes beyond the human factor. Its benefits have been examined recently in the healthcare system after redefining criteria to achieve its intended purpose (Simmons, 2001).

The US Department of Veterans Affairs' National Center for Patient Safety (NCPS) of the US Department of Veterans' Affairs, which developed a new root cause analysis model to be used in the healthcare system consisting of assigning a safety assessment code to prioritise errors and a human factor engineering approach for analysis, considered it essential to achieve safety in the healthcare system (Bagian *et al.*, 2002). The JCAHO defines root cause analysis as

> [A] process for identifying the most basic or causal factors that underlie variation in performance, including the occurrence of an adverse sentinel event. . . . The analysis identifies changes that could be made in systems and processes through either redesign or development of new systems and processes that would improve the level of performance and reduce the risk of a particular serious adverse event occurring in the future. Root cause analysis focuses primarily on systems and processes, not individual performance; the analysis progresses from special causes in clinical processes to common causes in organizational processes; and the analysis repeatedly digs deeper by asking 'why?' questions until no additional logical answer can be identified.
>
> Berry and Krizek (2000)

Tools have been developed to assist the conduction of root cause analysis. These tools could be paper-based templates or software programs. Table 3.5 is a description of the steps involved in root cause analysis as suggested by the NPSA in the UK.

The accident causation model

Also known as Reason's Swiss cheese model, this model has been applied in the aviation industry and in understanding the causes of medication errors. Reason (1998) explained that defence mechanisms in any organisation can be represented as slices of cheese. These might be engineered defences such as alarms, physical barriers, or individuals such as surgeons, pilots. Ideally, the slices of cheese should be intact, but in reality they have holes which, unlike the static holes of the Swiss cheese, are continuously changing in size, opening and closing. The holes represent active failures due to slips, lapses, mistakes and, rarely, violations conducted by individuals. They also represent latent conditions, more to do with organisational and procedural errors commonly made by managers, designers and builders. He added that under certain circumstances holes open up and line up together to permit the transition of an accident. He explained that such error-producing conditions can be classified as environmental factors, team factors, individual factors and factors related to the task carried out. The accident causation model is summarised in Figure 3.1.

Table 3.5 Description of the steps involved in root cause analysis

1. Classifying the incident	The NHS uses the 5×5 matrix with colour coding or textual descriptors
2. Setting the team	Includes experts, specialists and those who were in contact with the incident
3. Scoping the incident	Acute episodes analysed completely while chronic can be explored at any point where incident happened and worked backwards to track data
4. Data gathering	Sources of information are clinical staff, the patient and the carers, medical records, policies and procedures
5. Information mapping	Different templates such as timeline, tabular timeline or narrative chronology
6. Identifying problems	Done naturally at the gathering and mapping steps, problems noted as either care delivery problem or service delivery problem
7. Analysing problems for contributory factors	Using contributory factor framework, cause and effect method, tree diagram, barrier analysis and 'the five why's' technique. Each contributory factor identified in the analysis could be a causal factor or an influencing factor
8. Agreeing the root causes	This can be done using nominal group technique or brainstorming
9. Recommending and reporting	Actions should prevent or reduce the occurrence of an event resourced; they should be implemented and evaluated for effectiveness through barrier analysis

Application in the accident causation model

In this section, a real case is presented so that the accident causation model can be applied to identify the root cause of the errors (BBC News, 1999a–g).

Case: morphine injection fatal medication errors

Background

Baby LW was given a dose of morphine which was 100 times stronger than it should have been. The death certificate said Baby LW died from a brain disease and breathing difficulties.

Baby LW, who was born 7 weeks prematurely and had difficulty breathing, was given the morphine to sedate her. Dr HE (Senior House Officer) is alleged to have miscalculated the amount of morphine that

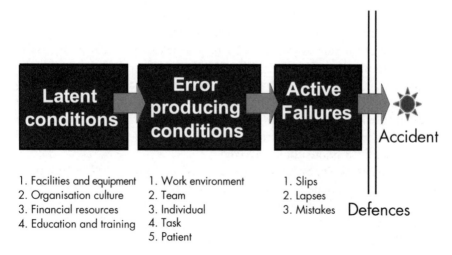

Figure 3.1 The accident causation model (ACM).

she needed by 100 times after writing the sum down on a piece of scrap paper.

The dosage should have been 0.15 mg, but was in fact 15 mg.

Dr VM (Senior Registrar) was given the morphine and reportedly failed to spot that the dosage was too high.

The inquest into the death recorded an open verdict. However, the coroner also criticised Dr HE for her lack of mathematical skills.

Nurses' evidence

Nurse SS said there had been 'pandemonium' in the hospital that day, and it was in that atmosphere that she had breached hospital protocol by signing the drugs register.

Nurse SS said: 'The baby looked so sick I thought at that stage the baby was going to die. Other babies were crying. There were visitors already in the unit and others entering. A baby of a drug addict mother was basically screaming, going through withdrawal. It was pandemonium, hectic.'

Nurse SS said: 'I asked Dr HE why she needed it [the second ampoule]. [Dr HE replied] there wasn't enough.' Nurse SS asked what Dr HE was giving. Dr HE said '156 micrograms'. Nurse said to Dr HE 'What are you giving?'. Then Dr HE picked up a calculator and did the calculation. Nurse SS read the figure on the calculator screen which said

1.5. Nurse SS thought she said 'That's not right, it's too much' but she was not quite sure of the words she said at that time.

One of the nurses (Sister BL) who was involved in caring for Baby LW before she died said: 'She [Baby LW] became so relaxed so suddenly. I asked him how much he had given her and he said 15 milligrams. I said she only required 100 micrograms per kilo of bodyweight. He looked shocked and said "Oh, you are right".'

About half an hour after Baby LW had received the overdose of morphine, Dr S (Consultant) arrived.

Another nurse, Sister JL, said Dr VM had given Dr S a summary of what had happened to Baby LW. Dr S then had to tell Baby LW's mother that her daughter was dying. Sister JL said Dr S told the parents that the baby had had a large dose of morphine, but she did not tell them the size of it or who gave it to her.

Family's evidence

The baby's father told the hearing that he and his wife only found out 16 months after the baby's death that she had been given the wrong dose of morphine. The father said: 'She [Dr S] just said "There has been a mistake. We overdosed on morphine and we have counter-acted it with an antidote". She just said it was a large amount. She said "I have got to admit that I overdosed on morphine but I rectified it straight away".'

The father said Dr S did not tell them the extent of the overdose or who gave it to her. The parents assumed that it was Dr S who administered the morphine and did not find out the truth until much later.

Consultant's evidence

Dr S said: 'I listened to the sequence of events as told to me by Dr VM and I thought that the features of her illness were of respiratory problems; I had experience of a morphine overdose just two months before in a similar situation. A baby was given 10 times too much but the mistake was spotted almost immediately and nothing happened to the baby. So I did not think 100 times morphine equalled death. I thought we had counteracted the morphine and the problem was respiratory.'

Dr S said that this was why she did not mention morphine on the death certificate, which she instructed Dr VM to fill out. Dr S also denied that she tried to mislead Louise's parents about the overdose, but admitted that she had made an error of judgement by not reporting the death to the coroner immediately.

Senior Registrar's evidence

Dr VM said he trusted Dr HE because he had worked with her before. Dr VM described Dr HE as a 'very easy person to work with, very energetic, efficient, good at taking histories and assessing situations'.

Police evidence

Dr HE said that she had only been on the ward for 2 months as part of her training to be a GP, and it was the first time that she had prepared a morphine dose for a baby.

Analysis

When we apply the accident causation model, the following key root causes will be identified.

Latent condition

1. Equipment – morphine ampoule was designed for adults; therefore the concentration is too high for neonates
2. Organisation culture:
    (a) Another baby was given 10 times morphine overdose 2 months ago, but the organisation did not learn from the mistake and implement changes in procedure.
    (b) The procedure of informing relatives about the errors was inadequate.
3. Education and training:
    (a) The coroner criticised Dr HE for her lack of mathematical skills.
    (b) Dr HE said that she had only been on the ward for 2 months as part of her training to be a GP, and it was the first time that she had prepared a morphine dose for a baby

Error-producing condition

1. Work environment:
    (a) Paediatric ward is at higher risk than other wards.
    (b) Nurse SS said that there had been 'pandemonium' in the hospital that day.

2. Team:
    (a) Nurses and doctors were not working as a team to communicate the important message. Nurse SS knew the dosage was not right but failed to communicate this important message.
    (b) Dr VM said that he trusted Dr HE because he had worked with her before, but without assessing the quality of the work.
3. Individual:
    (a) See education and training about Dr HE.
    (b) Nurse SS had breached hospital protocol by signing the drugs register.
4. Task – see education and training about Dr HE.
5. Patient – a premature baby is always at high risk from medication errors.

Active failure

1. Mistakes – Dr HE made the calculation errors.
2. Lapses – Dr VM did not check the dose before giving

Active 'defences' (interventions) can be put in place to prevent future tenfold calculation errors (e.g. good medication error reporting and analysis system, double-checking system, and better training and supervision).

Suggestions to prevent medication errors in children

During the last few years many different guidelines and recommendations have been published by professional organisations, government and researchers on prevention of medication errors. The following is a summary of some important suggestions produced by the American Academy of Pediatrics Committee on Drugs and Committee on Hospital Cares, Institute for Safe Medication Practices and the Pediatric Pharmacy Advocacy Group (Levine *et al.*, 2001; Stucky, 2003). Readers will find that many of these are 'common sense' suggestions.

Prescribing

- Prescribers should not prescribe paediatric medications if they are not familiar with either the drug or paediatrics.

- Prescribers should check drug allergies, interactions and contra-indications and note these on the drug chart.
- Prescribers should confirm that the patient's weight is correct and write the weight on each drug chart.
- Weight-based dose should not exceed the recommended adult dose.
- Prescribers should write legible prescriptions.

Calculation

- Prescribers should write out each step of a calculation for double-checking.
- The calculation should be double-checked by other staff.

Administration

- Nurses/clinicians should check the drug, dose and patient identity before administration.
- Any unusual volumes or dosages should be verified with pre-scribers.
- Nurses/clinicians should listen to the patient or parent or caregiver attentively, answer questions, and double-check with the pre-scribers when a query arises as to whether a drug should be admin-istered.

Hospital environment

- An adequate number of qualified staff and a suitable work environ-ment for safe and effective use of medicines should be provided.
- Staff should also have sufficient training and continuous education in the use of paediatric medications.
- Equipment (e.g. infusion pump) and measurement systems should be standardised to remove much of the risks of calculation errors as well as to reduce the time required for dose calculation.
- Barriers to medication error reporting should be eliminated and a non-punitive culture encouraged. This will allow a well-developed medication error reporting system to be developed to collect vital information for root cause analysis and risk assessment.
- Hospitals should develop and maintain a process for informing families of errors and feedback information to staff.

References

Bagian J P, Gosbee J, Lee C Z, Williams L, McKnight S D, Mannos D M (2002). The Veterans Affairs root cause analysis system in action. *Jt Comm J Qual Improv* 28: 531–545.

BBC News (2004). Pills mistake 'could be fatal'. A baby in Bristol was twice dispensed heart drugs more than 10 times stronger than doctors had prescribed. http://news.bbc.co.uk/1/hi/england/bristol/3629907.stm.

BBC News (1999a). Doctors accused over baby overdose. 19 April. http://news.bbc.co.uk/1/hi/health/323175.stm.

BBC News (1999b). Nurse questioned overdose doctor's judgement. 20 April. http://news.bbc.co.uk/1/hi/health/323959.stm.

BBC News (1999c). Overdose doctor cleared. 20 April. http://news.bbc.co.uk/1/hi/health/324382.stm.

BBC News (1999d). Weeping doctor apologises to parents. 21 April. http://news.bbc.co.uk/1/hi/health/325416.stm.

BBC News (1999e). Consultant doubted overdose killed baby. 22 April. http://news.bbc.co.uk/1/hi/health/326000.stm.

BBC News (1999f). Overdose doctors cleared. 23 April. http://news.bbc.co.uk/1/hi/health/326656.stm.

BBC News (1999g). An easy mistake to make. 23 April. http://news.bbc.co.uk/hi/english/health/newsid_326000/326947.stm.

Berry K, Krizek B (2000). Root cause analysis in response to a 'near miss'. *J Healthcare Qual* 22: 16–18.

Blum K V, Abel S R, Urbanski C J, Pierce J M (1988). Medication error prevention by pharmacists. *Am J Hosp Pharm* 45: 1902–1903.

Bruce J, Wong I C K (2001). Parenteral drug administration errors by nursing staff on an acute medical admissions ward during day duty. *Drug Safety* 24: 855–862.

Cimino M A, Kirschbaum MS, Brodsky L, Shaha S H (2004). Assessing medication prescribing errors in pediatric intensive care units. *Pediatr Crit Care Med* 5: 124–132.

Cousins D, Clarkson A, Conroy S, Choonara I (2002). Medication errors in children – an eight year review using press reports. *Paediatr Perinatal Drug Ther* 5: 52–58.

Cowley E, Williams R, Cousins D (2001). Medication errors in children: a descriptive summary of medication error reports submitted to the United States Pharmacopoeia. *Curr Ther Res* 62: 627–640.

Dean B, Schachter M, Vincent C, Barber N D (2002). Prescribing errors in hospital inpatients – their incidence and clinical significance. *Qual Safety Health Care* 11: 340–344.

DeRosier J, Stalhandske E, Bagian J P, Nudell T (2002). Using health care failure mode and effect analysis: the VA National Center for Patient Safety's prospective risk analysis system. *Jt Comm J Qual Improv* 28: 248–267.

Folli H L, Poole R L, Benitz W E, Russo J C (1987). Medication error prevention by clinical pharmacists in two children's hospitals. *Pediatrics* 79: 718–722.

Fontan J E, Maneglier V, Nguyen V X, Loirat C, Brion F (2003). Medication errors in hospitals: computerized unit dose drug dispensing system versus ward stock distribution system. *Pharmacy World and Science* 25: 112–117.

Ghaleb M A, Wong I C K (2006). Medication errors in children. *Arch Dis Child Educ Pract* 91: 20.

Ghaleb M A, Barber N, Dean Franklin B, Wong I C K (2005). What constitutes a prescribing error in paediatrics – a Delphi study. *Qual Saf Health Care* 14: 352–357.

Gothard A M, Dade J P, Murphy K, Mellor E J (2004). Using error theory in the pharmacy dispensary can reduce accidents. *Pharm Pract* 14: 44–48.

Herout P M, Erstad B L (2004). Medication errors involving continuously infused medications in a surgical intensive care unit. *Crit Care Med* 32: 428–432.

Kaushal R, Bates D W, Landrigan C, *et al.* (2001). Medication errors and adverse drug events in pediatric inpatients. *JAMA* 285: 2114–2120.

Kohn L T, Corrigan J M, Donaldson M S (1999). *To Err is Human: Building a Safer Health System.* Washington DC: Institute of Medicine National Academy Press.

Kozer E, Scolnik D, Macpherson A, Keays T, Shi K, Luk T, Koren G (2002). Variables associated with medication errors in pediatric emergency medicine. *Pediatrics* 110: 737–742.

Levine S R, Cohen M R, Blanchard N R, *et al.* (2001). Guidelines for preventing medication errors in pediatrics. *J Pediatr Pharmacol Ther* 6: 426–442.

Marino B L, Reinhardt K, Eichelberger W J, Steingard R (2000). Prevalence of errors in a pediatric hospital medication system: Implication for error proofing. *Outcomes Manag Nurs Pract* 4: 129–135.

National Patient Safety Agency. RCA Foundation Training and RCA toolkit. http://81.144.177.110/web/display. content Id=2665.

Nixon P, Dhillon S (1996). Medication errors in paediatrics. *Progress in Practice: UKCPA Autumn Symposium,* 18–19.

Paton J, Wallace J (1997). Medication errors. *Lancet* 349: 959–960.

Reason J (1998). Achieving a safe culture: theory and practice. *Work Stress* 12: 293–306.

Ross L M, Wallace J, Paton J Y (2000). Medication errors in a paediatric teaching hospital in the UK: five years operational experience. *Arch Dis Child* 83: 492–497.

Schneider M-P, Cotting J, Pannatier A (1998). Evaluation of nurses' errors associated in the preparation and administration of medication in a pediatric intensive care unit. *Pharm World Sci* 20: 178–182.

Selbst S M, Fein J A, Osterhoudt K, Ho W (1999). Medication errors in a pediatric emergency department. *Pediatr Emerg Care* 15: 1–4.

Simmons J C (2001). How root-cause analysis can improve patient safety. *Qual Lett Healthcare Leaders* 13: 2–12.

Stucky E R (2003). American Academy of Pediatrics Committee on Drugs; American Academy of Pediatrics Committee on Hospital Care. Prevention of medication errors in the pediatric inpatient setting. *Pediatrics* 112: 431–436.

Weinberg N (2001). Using performance measures to identify plans of action to improve care. *Jt Comm J Qual Improv* 27: 683–688.

Wilson D G, McArtney R G, Newcombe R G, *et al.* (1998). Medication errors in paediatric practice: insights from a continuous quality improvement approach. *Eur J Pediatr* 157: 769–774.

Wong I C K, Ghaleb M, Dean Franklin B, Barber N (2004). Incidence and nature of dosing errors in paediatric medications – A systematic review. *Drug Safety* 27: 661–670.

4

Paediatric formulations in practice

Catherine Tuleu

Introduction

It has been internationally recognised that children are at risk when they are administered unsuitable medicines. In many cases, the only medicines available have not been clinically tested for safety, efficacy and quality in relation to the age group for which they are used. Problems resulting from a lack of suitably adapted medicines for children include inaccurate dosing, increased risk of adverse reactions (including death), ineffective treatment (under-dosing), unavailability to children of therapeutic advances (modified-release forms) and extemporaneous formulations for children that may exhibit poor or inconsistent bioavailability, low quality and low safety.

Children represent a vulnerable group with anatomical, developmental, physiological and psychological differences from adults, making age- and development-related research in relation to the specific needs of children particularly complex. This is especially true when it comes to designing appropriate dosage forms for such a heterogeneous population. Developmental changes, especially in early childhood, affecting bioavailability, pharmacokinetics, pharmacodynamics and pharmacogenomics, will influence the choice of optimum medicines in various age groups. Non-biological considerations such as motor and psychological development, ability to coordinate and willingness to cooperate, health status (acute or long-term disease), geographical and sociocultural background, will also influence the choice of dosage form for optimal administration in heterogeneous age groups. Compliance issues are even further complicated by the fact that a third contributor (parents, caregivers, nurses) is also involved.

This chapter will discuss drug handling in paediatric practice, general considerations in extemporaneous dispensing for children, the suitability of excipients, and the potential of the main administration routes and corresponding dosage forms in paediatrics.

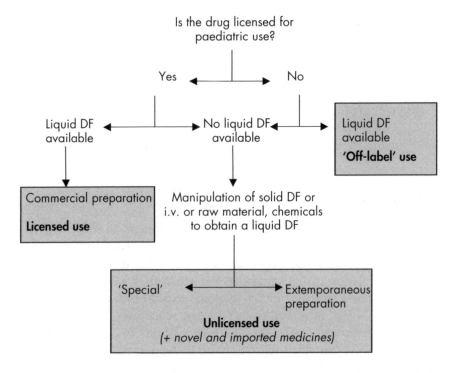

Figure 4.1 Decision pathway for providing oral doses to children for whom whole tablets/capsules are unsuitable (DF = dosage form, i.v. = intravenous). Adapted from Standing and Tuleu (2005), with permission of the authors.

The use of off-licensed and unlicensed medicines

Before any medicine is authorised for adult use, the product must have undergone clinical testing to ensure that it is safe, effective and of high quality. This is not the case with all medicines for hospitalised children as, depending on specialty, between 15 and 80% are not licensed for purpose (termed 'off-license' or 'off-label' [OL] in the USA) or have not been licensed at all (termed 'unlicensed' [UL]). This is also the case in the community but possibly to a lesser extent.

Using medicines that are not licensed means that there is limited available evidence on safety, quality and efficacy, and a potentially increased risk of adverse drug reaction. In addition to a lack of systematically compiled evidence for the use of UL and OL medicines, many are available only as monolithic solid dosage forms. As dosing is often based on body weight, only a proportion of a solid dosage form has to be given, which can be difficult to achieve. Figure 4.1 summarises the options available to administer oral medicines to children who cannot swallow whole solid dosage forms.

Ideally, if there is no appropriate dosage form for a drug, another drug with the same therapeutic spectrum but adequate formulation, such as liquid, effervescent, dispersible tablets, is recommended in accordance with the prescriber.

The term 'OL medicine' may be used to describe a drug in an adequate dosage form for administration to children (e.g. liquid formulation) but which is being used outside the specification terms of the product licence (or marketing authorisation). For example, in the UK, there is an adult licensed liquid preparation of atenolol but it is not licensed for children. OL may also be given:

- by an unlicensed route of administration (e.g. lorazepam injection given orally)
- for an unlicensed indication (e.g. sildenafil for pulmonary hypertension)
- at an unlicensed dose (e.g. salbutamol nebules are licensed for adult use at up to 40 mg a day but can be given to children at up to 60 mg a day)
- outside the age limits stated in the licence (e.g. diazepam rectal solution, although not licensed for children under 1 year, is used in infants)
- even if contraindicated for use in children (e.g. aspirin used in Kawasaki's disease and some cardiac patients but generally not recommended for children because of its association with Reye's syndrome).

UL medicines are medicines under an unlicensed dosage form obtained after manipulation of the original dosage form (e.g. crushing/cutting tablets, extemporaneous preparations, 'special'). Sometimes the drug itself may have no licence at all (e.g. chemicals used in metabolic diseases, such as betaine to treat homocystinuria, and novel medicines). Imported medicines become unlicensed in the country into which they are imported.

In general, it is not necessary to obtain the explicit consent from children, parents or carers to prescribe or administer UL or OL medicines. Nevertheless, a clear explanation should be given.

When a company supplies a product for which no product licence exists, it is usually supplied on a named patient basis, meaning that the consultant's name, patient's name and the conditions that the drug is being used to treat are all recorded.

In the UK, section 10 of the Medicines Act and Regulations (1968) provides an exemption that enables doctors to:

- prescribe unlicensed medicines
- use specially prepared, imported or supplied unlicensed products in certain patients, on a named basis
- use medicines that are not authorised to be marketed, in clinical trials, following approval of the trial (novel medicines) by the local regulators (Medicines and Healthcare products Regulatory Agency [MHRA] in the UK)
- use or advise the use of licensed medicines for indications, or in doses, or by routes of administration, outside the recommendation of the licence
- override the warnings and the precautions given in the licence.

This varies among countries, and the above applies only in the UK.

Extemporaneous dispensing

More and more clinical trials in children are taking place and are improving the availability of ready-made specific paediatric drug delivery systems. Moreover, from the perspective of the new European Union regulations on medicines for children (European Commission, 2006), the number of trials will increase in the future. Meanwhile, extemporaneous dispensing, even though it should remain the last resort, is still an important activity for paediatric pharmacists and carers (Yeung *et al.*, 2004).

Ideally, extemporaneous products are prepared from pure drugs (or less suitably from chemicals) but, more frequently, commercial dosage forms intended for adults are manipulated into a suitable form for administration to children. They should be prepared in registered premises (pharmacy, hospital, health centre) under the supervision of a pharmacist and in accordance with a prescription for administration to a particular patient or in anticipation of such a prescription. These manipulations come under the heading of magistral (extemporaneous) preparations. 'Specials' have a similar status but are made in larger volumes by licensed manufacturers (licence issued by the MHRA in the UK), which include suitably licensed hospital units. However, these products are not always subjected to full quality assurance.

In practice, many extemporaneous preparations are made by nurses/carers at home or at the bedside. This non-'special' extemporaneous dispensing carries a greater risk as very little risk assessment or risk management is in place. Frequent pharmaceutical problems encountered with such preparations are their lack of validation and standardisation, their lack of stability data and the lack of proof of dose uniformity. Dosing accuracy, reproducibility and bioavailability, due to a general lack of information and peer-reviewed research in this field, are major problems. The suitability of excipients susceptible to age-related toxicity will be discussed in another section of this chapter.

Solid dosage forms

For patient acceptability, oral drug delivery is the preferred route of administration. Tablets and capsules are the most popular way of delivering a drug for oral use. They are convenient for patients who can swallow them because they deliver an accurate dose, they are compact and economically mass produced by the pharmaceutical industry, and the delivery profile of the drug can be modified. Solid dosage forms are virtually free from taste and major stability problems encountered with liquids. Nevertheless, their main disadvantage for children is the non-flexibility of dose and some children's, especially the very young, difficulty or inability to swallow them whole.

The practice of crushing tablets or opening capsules and adding the powder to water, a palatable drink or food is frequent with children and problems often arise, mainly linked to the quantification of dose administered. Manufacturers' advice should be sought for compatibility of drinks and food and any known effect on bioavailability. A mortar and pestle are recommended to crush tablets but devices for containing, crushing and dispersing the tablets should be used outside the dispensary by parents and carers (Figure 4.2).

Dose inaccuracy occurs when unscored tablets are cut to obtain the required dose or to facilitate swallowing: the weight of a split tablet can range from 50% to 150% of the actual half-tablet weight (Teng *et al.*, 2002) and accuracy does not seem to be improved by using commercially available tablet-cutter devices (Breitkreutz *et al.*, 1999) similar to the one shown in Figure 4.3. Some tablets (enteric-coated, multilayered tablets, modified-release tablets) cannot be manipulated without affecting the release properties and possible therapeutic effects, unless especially stated by the manufacturer (Tuleu *et al.*, 2005). Splitting tablets into segments is not recommended with narrow therapeutic index drugs, potent or cytotoxic drugs, or small tablets.

Tablets are often crushed or capsules opened and dispersed in a small volume of water to give a fractional dose with a syringe. Even if

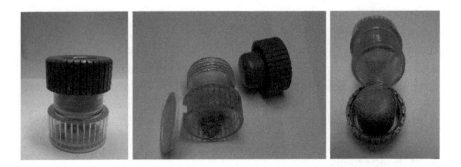

Figure 4.2 Tablet cutter.

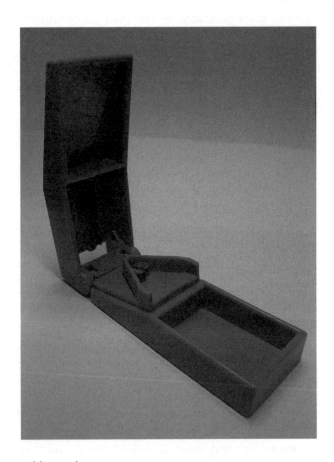

Figure 4.3 Tablet crusher.

the drug itself is soluble, the mixture should be shaken prior to measuring the dose as extraction from excipients may not be complete. Filtering should not be undertaken unless it has been established that the active drug will not be removed. In the case of insoluble drugs the sedimentation process can provide highly variable dosing, especially if the dose (volume) is small. Moreover, taste becomes a problem once the drug and the excipients are in solution.

If no alternative is available, fractional doses can be prepared by diluting powdered tablets or capsules with suitable common excipients, such as lactose or starch, and repacking them into sachets or empty capsules using a hand-filling machine. It is important that uniformity of dose distribution and incompatibility or stability of new single units can be compromised and should be checked with appropriate pharmacopoeial monographs.

In order to adjust the dose, splitting suppositories, like splitting tablets, assumes initial uniform distribution of the drug, although this is not a pharmacopoeial requirement. Nevertheless, due to the solidification step during the manufacturing process, dose uniformity is much more uncertain. Moreover, the shapes of suppositories do not facilitate halving them and the resulting shape may not be optimal for rectal insertion. In any case, they should be cut lengthwise in order to decrease dosage errors.

There are no transdermal patches commercially available for paediatric use but in certain therapeutic situations they might be applied to children's skin as described in a few research articles (caffeine, theophylline, oestrogen, testosterone, fentanyl, hyoscine). The dose being proportional to the surface area of the patch, manipulation of a matrix or adhesive-type patch to adapt the dose can be achieved by cutting it. In order to adapt the dose of a reservoir-type patch, it is partially covered with a non-diffusible membrane in practice but not cut. Great care has to be taken as it is an empirical procedure and, when cutting patches, it can be difficult to assess the area loaded with drug or it can lead to drug instability when exposed to the atmosphere. Manufacturers' advice and expertise should be sought.

Liquid dosage forms

If no adequate dosage form is available, it is possible to use oral liquids rectally, eye drops in the ear or a sometimes costly injectable solution orally (e.g. clonidine) and, less frequently, by respiratory routes (e.g. gentamicin, vancomycin). Doses may need to be adapted due to differing bioavailability by a different route (kinetics of absorption, extensive first-pass metabolism). Prodrugs might not be activated if the route of administration is different (e.g. cefuroxime axetil, enalapril maleate). Stomach residence might alter the drug and its solubility (e.g. acetazolamide sodium/acetazolamide, sodium folinate/folic acid) or degrade the drug (e.g. proton pump inhibitors such as omeprazole). Injectable drugs are commonly formulated as solutions. Most solutions are aqueous, although non-aqueous solutions (propylene glycol, glycerol, oils, liposomes, etc.) are also available to increase drug solubility or stability or to modify the release when injected.

Other additives such as antimicrobial agents, antioxidants, buffers and tonicity-adjusting agents can be included in injection formulations and it is the responsibility of the pharmacist to check that all excipients and adjuvants are suitable (benzyl alcohol, ethanol, sulfites, sodium content, etc.). Nevertheless, one is left with a difficult choice over excipients, either those for which toxicity is known and therefore predictable, or those with safety profiles that have not been established in children (see under Critical excipients, page 55). The pH and osmolarity of the preparation must also be checked before administration by another route.

To achieve an appropriate strength, it is sometimes necessary to dilute the commercial preparations. Not only can physical and chemical stability be compromised but dilution may also render preservatives ineffective. For complex formulations in particular the suitability of the diluent must be assessed prior to manipulation. When drugs are unstable in solution, they are usually formulated as dry powders for reconstitution with an appropriate diluent (water) and most paediatric doses will require withdrawal of a dose volume that is different to the total volume after reconstitution. This can lead to medication errors (Wong *et al.*, 2004).

The most frequent method used to prepare oral liquids remains the use of ground tablets and capsule contents mixed with a vehicle. For cytotoxic drugs, antibiotics or sensitising agents, the same rules apply but procedures must be carried out under conditions that protect the operator from exposure to the drug and prevent contamination. Standard procedures relating to the compounding of cytotoxic drugs should be followed.

Some vehicles are commercially available (Table 4.1).

Ora-Plus is an oral vehicle suited for use in the preparation of oral, non-soluble (suspended), aqueous dosage forms, commercialised by Paddock Laboratories Inc. in North America. Ora-Plus is a blank vehicle

Table 4.1 Suspension vehicles and flavouring agents commercially available

Ingredients[a]	Ora-Plus	Ora-Sweet	Ora-Sweet SF	Ora-Blend	Ora-Blend SF
Microcrystalline cellulose (%)	<1	✗	✗	<1	<1
Sodium carboxy-methylcellulose (%)	<1	✗	✗	<1	<1
Sucrose (%)	✗	54	✗	>10	✗
Glycerol (%)	✗	5	10	<10	<10
Sorbitol (%)	✗	4	9	<10	<10
Sodium saccharin (%)	✗	✗	0.1	✗	<1
Xanthan gum (%)	<1	✗	✓	<1	<1
Carrageenan (%)	<1	✗	✗	<1	<1
Flavouring agent (%)	✗	<1	✓	<1	<1
Citric acid (%)	<0.1	<1	✓	<1	<1
Sodium phosphate (%)	<0.1	<1	✗	<1	<1
Sodium citrate (%)	✗	✗	✓	✗	<1
Simethicone (%)	<0.1	✗	✗	<1	<1
Methylparaben (%)	<0.1	<1	✓	<1	<1
Propylparaben (%)	✗	✗	✓	✗	<1
Potassium sorbate (%)	<0.1	<1	✓	<1	<1
Purified water (%)	97	✓	✓	>10	>10

From Paddock Laboratories Inc. (2003).
✓ when the ingredient is present in the preparation at a percentage not specified in the Material Safety Data Sheet.

containing an antifoaming agent and preservatives. Ora-Sweet and its sugar-free equivalent (Ora-Sweet SF) are syrup vehicles, alcohol free and citrus–berry flavoured, which may be used alone or in conjunction with suspending agents to impart flavour and sweetness. They both contain preservatives and are buffered to a slightly acidic pH (around pH 4). They have been used in many formulation and stability studies published in North America (Nahata and Hipple, 2003; Paddocks Laboratories Inc., 2003), often in a 50/50 ratio of Ora-Plus to Ora-Sweet or Ora-Sweet SF. The corresponding 50/50 preparations are now available under the names Ora-Blend and Ora-Blend SF.

Nevertheless, simpler suspending and flavouring agents can also be prepared at the dispensary (e.g. methylcellulose 1%, or other celluloses such as hypromellose, microcrystalline cellulose, sodium carboxy-methylcellulose at 1–2%, xanthan gels, pharmacopoeial syrups, or mixtures of the above). In some formulations suspending agents may not be required, for example, when it is known that the drug is soluble

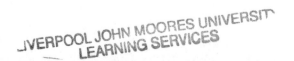

in the vehicle. The use of syrup, glycerol or sorbitol as simple suspending agents may be adequate. However, other agents might often be required: alternative co-solvents (ethanol, propylene glycol), wetting agents to help suspend crushed tablets or capsules' contents (Polysorbate 80 at 0.5% v/v, ethanol at 5–15% v/v), buffer systems to optimise pH for drug stability and/or activity of the preservative system (benzoates). Citric acid, sodium benzoate, benzoic acid or parabens is often added as a preservative. The effectiveness of antimicrobial preservatives is reduced by chemical degradation, binding interactions with macro-molecules or upon dilution, for example when a commercial vehicle is mixed with a non-preserved in-house vehicle. For this reason, mixtures should not be stored for prolonged periods without appropriate testing to validate the shelf-life. For small-scale operations preparation of the suspending agent at the time of dispensing is recommended.

Excipients contained in the original dosage form also have to be taken into account and can decrease the product's appearance (insolubles) or even reduce the drug stability. The end-product is therefore a complex and not well-defined admixture of numerous components. Ideally, it should be prepared with the pure active pharmaceutical ingredient when possible.

In an attempt to provide some guidance, a few publications describing extemporaneous dispensing have been compiled (Nahata and Hipple, 2003; Woods, 2001) and should be referred to as well as peer-reviewed journals.

Usually the information the reader can find is:

- Formulas
- Method of manufacture, although there is often a lack of important detail (e.g. clear protocols for the homogenisation step in the preparation of suspensions) impairing their reproducibility
- Special mention (if any) regarding its use
- Conditions of storage and shelf-life, often based only on chemical stability without addressing possible physical or microbiological spoilage that may occur during the use of the product accompanied by a published peer-reviewed reference if available.

Semi-solid dosage forms

Proprietary alternatives are often available, so compounding of semi-solids is not an extensive activity in paediatrics. Standard compounding conditions apply. Aqueous creams are prone to microbial growth which is often counteracted by adding preservatives. When creams are mixed or diluted, apart from the risk of introducing microorganisms, the preservative system can be inactivated through incompatibility, dilution or changes in partition coefficient. On the rare occasion where compounding is necessary, a short shelf-life should be assigned.

Stability issues

The main causes for the limited time for which medicines can be kept are:

- Loss of drug (by degradation)
- Loss of vehicle (by evaporation)
- Loss of uniformity (by caking of a suspension)
- Change of organoleptic characters (appearance)
- Change of bioavailability
- Appearance of degradation product that might be irritant or toxic.

Dispensing may inadvertently shorten the shelf-life of a product in view of its susceptibility not only to chemical challenge but also to physical or microbiological challenge, which may be significant during actual use of the product. Extemporaneous preparations are often given arbitrary shelf-lives or based on published information for a particular formulation. The term 'freshly' and 'recently' prepared are used by the pharmacopoeias to describe preparations that are respectively made 24 hours before their issue for use and discarded 4 weeks after issue when stored at 15–25°C. Where a shelf-life of 28 days or more is assigned, consideration should be given to producing these products in a licensed manufacturing unit. A conservative approach must be adopted when assigning a longer expiry date because of lack of information on drug stability or limitations in either the design or the conclusions of a published report. Also, it may be impractical to reproduce entirely the controlled conditions of an experiment in clinical or domiciliary settings. The adequacy of the reference stability testing must be ensured.

Physical stability

Dispersed systems such as suspensions can lead to physical instability which can be simply measured by the rate of sedimentation of solids undissolved in the preparation. The formulator should ensure that the suspended material does not settle too rapidly; the particles that do settle to the bottom of the container must not form a hard mass, but should be readily dispersed into a uniform mixture when the container is shaken. In practice, adequate testing should be undertaken when establishing the shelf-life. This includes the ease of redispersion in parallel with the uniformity of dose. Viscosity of preparations is also a critical physical parameter and should be monitored as changes can affect the redispersion and pourability of the preparation, and impair dosing. Temperature (refrigeration or evaporation of volatile solvent) can affect viscosity and induce precipitation of actives or excipients such as preservatives, which can lead to erratic dosing or affect the quality of the preparation. If the drug itself is in suspension, particle size can affect the uniformity of the drug content since large particles settle faster than smaller ones. Particle size of suspensions may increase during storage as a result of sedimentation, aggregation or crystal growth which can occur due to Ostwald ripening, fluctuation in storage temperature or changes in polymorphic form.

Measurement of particle size distribution of suspensions may also affect the dissolution and bioavailability of certain drugs. Larger particles tend to have lower solubility and slower dissolution rates; consequently these particles have lower bioavailability. It is especially significant for poorly soluble drugs for which dissolution is the limiting step in absorption. For example, the absorptions of griseofulvin, nitrofurantoin and spironolactone are significantly influenced by the particle size of the drugs.

Chemical stability

The most common reactions leading to chemical instability of pharmaceuticals are hydrolysis, oxidation and reduction.

In the solid state, access to light and oxygen can catalyse oxidation and photochemical degradation. Access to moisture can induce hydrolysis. For sensitive drugs, lighting, temperature and humidity control should be adequate during manufacture and storage to limit degradation of ingredients. Containers, packaging, conditions of storage and labelling should also be adapted to the product. Usually drugs in the solid state or in suspension are considered more stable than drugs in solution.

In the liquid state, temperature and pH are major determinants that affect the hydrolysis rate. Trace metals and oxidising agents can also catalyse the degradation phenomenon. For hydrolysable drugs, the pH of optimum stability is on the acid side (pH 5–6). Buffering agents are often used in extemporaneous formulation to avoid variation of the pH upon storage. Antioxidants can be added to divert the oxidative process. Keeping liquids refrigerated slows down chemical reaction rate and bacterial growth, but could change the thickness of the vehicle, making resuspension and dosing difficult.

Microbiological stability

Microbiological growth can occur in aqueous medicines and contamination could lead to spoilage or toxicity. The effect on the organoleptic characters of the preparation can range from turbidity to bad odour and taste. The presence of microorganisms and their metabolites can more seriously impair the chemical stability and the drug solubility by affecting the pH. As most preservatives have optimised activity at a specific pH, a change in pH could affect the preservative system efficacy of the liquid. The use of contaminated ingredients or packaging, incorrect storage or unhygienic use of the product will also have an effect. This aspect of stability studies of extemporaneous preparations is often wrongly ignored.

Critical excipients

Formulation of liquids usually requires more excipients, in both type and quantity, than for solid dosage forms. They must be carefully selected in paediatric preparations because of possible pharmacological actions or toxic effects. Dose-related adverse effects of excipients are of particular concern in the preterm, low-birthweight neonate and infant due to immaturity of hepatic and renal function in this population. The following is not an exhaustive list but is intended to raise awareness of susceptible excipients to be used in paediatric medication. More emphasis is put on additional agents than on vehicles such as sweeteners and preservatives as they are of particular importance in paediatric liquid formulation and often not extensively taught at undergraduate levels.

In the European Union (EU), there are lists of approved additives, designated 'E' numbers as described in Table 4.2. The E stands for EC (European Community) and these ingredients have been tested for safety (allergenicity) and passed for use in the EU. Numbers that are not prefixed with an E may be allowed in the UK, for example, but may not have been passed for use in all EU countries. In the USA a different system is used which includes numbers instead. Therefore, for formulation purposes, the up-to-date lists of permitted flavouring and

Table 4.2 E colours and food additives classification

Additives	E numbers
Colours	100–181
Preservatives	200–290
Acids, antioxidants, mineral salts	300–390
Vegetal gums, emulsifiers, stabilisers, etc.	400–485, 500–585
Flavour enhancers	620–640
Miscellaneous (contains sweeteners)	>900

colouring agents should be consulted to choose acceptable additives in the country where the product is intended for use.

Vehicle composition

After water, ethanol is most commonly used in the formulation of oral liquids and is not without risk of acute overdose or chronic intoxication in children. There are still many extemporaneous and commercial preparations containing ethanol as co-solvents administered to children. Adverse effects to the central nervous system because of high blood–brain barrier permeability in children are reported, along with drug interactions linked with acute or chronic exposure. In the USA, the limits are set to a maximum of 10% alcohol in products for 12 year olds and over, a maximum of 5% alcohol in products intended for children aged 6–12 years and less than 0.5% alcohol content in products intended for children under 6 years of age. Nevertheless, further long-term research is needed to evaluate safety when this excipient is present in the drug formulation.

Propylene glycol (propane-1,2-diol), used in the formulation of lipid-soluble oral, topical and intravenous drugs (phenytoin, diazepam, digoxin and vitamins), is a less viscous liquid and a better solvent than glycerol, but practically tasteless. It has been widely demonstrated to cause osmotic laxative effects and contact dermatitis, and to increase the risk of serum hyperosmolality with a marked osmolar gap, lactic acidosis, seizures and cardiac arrhythmias when the patients received high-dose, long-term administration. Concern about propylene glycol toxicity prompted the World Health Organization (WHO) to establish a maximum daily intake limit of 25 mg/kg per day, although there is no known toxic dose. Propylene glycol toxicity is a potentially life-threatening iatrogenic complication (Wilson *et al.*, 2005). Propylene

Table 4.3 Selected food hypersensitivity and medication errors

Food	Medication
Egg	Fat emulsion, influenza vaccine, interferon alfa-n3, MM and MMR vaccines, propofol, verteporfin, yellow fever vaccine
Fish	Protamine
Iodine	Amiodarone, potassium iodide
Milk protein	Cefditoren pivoxil
Papaya	Crotalidae polyvalent immune Fab, digoxin immune Fab (ovine)
Peanut oil	Dimercaprol, ipratropium MDI, micronised progesterone in oil, soy isoflavones
Sesame oil	Dronabinol, fluphenazine decanoate, fat emulsion, haloperidol decanoate, nandrolone decanoate
Soy lecithin	Liposomal doxorubicin, fat emulsion, ipratropium MDI, propofol, soy isoflavone

MDI, metered dose inhaler; MMR, measles, mumps, rubella.
Adapted from Hofer *et al.* (2003) with permission of Harvey Whitney Books Co.

glycol is a racemic mixture of two optical isomers. L-Propylene glycol is dehydrogenated to L-lactic acid, a physiological intermediate, while D-propylene glycol gives rise to D-lactate, which is only slowly metabolised by the mitochondrial D-lactate dehydrogenase. Metabolic acidosis could be an important factor in nervous system complications (seizures) (Savolainen, 2005). It is not recommended in children below the age of 4 years as they have a limited metabolic pathway (alcohol dehydrogenase).

Oil formulations are not recommended for paediatric use because they are unpleasant to ingest and their use has been associated with diminished nutrient and vitamin absorption, with anal leakage and pruritus. They are especially unsuitable for nasal drop formulation as inadvertent aspiration has caused inflammatory and fibrotic changes in the lungs due to the inhalation of various fatty substances (lipid pneumonia).

Surfactants such as polysorbates may be used as solubilising agents. Polysorbate 80 has been associated with the E-Ferol syndrome (thrombocytopenia, renal dysfunction, hepatomegaly, cholestasis, ascites, hypotension and metabolic acidosis) in low-birthweight infants when used as a solubiliser aid in parenteral preparations.

Selected food hypersensitivity and medication interaction mainly due to one or more excipients may also preclude use of certain medications as listed in Table 4.3.

Sweetening agents

Sweeteners are commonly included in paediatric formulations to increase palatability and mask an unpleasant taste. Table 4.4 shows the relative sweetness of all the sweeteners discussed in this section.

Many oral solutions are sweetened with carbohydrates such as sucrose and glucose. Sucrose is a covalently bonded glucose and fructose residue, linked by a $(1{\rightarrow}2)\alpha\beta$-glycosidic bond. It is the most common sweetener, produced by concentrating the sugar from sugarcane or sugar beet juice, although it has been displaced by some other sweeteners such as glucose syrups or combinations of functional ingredients and high-intensity sweeteners. Sucrose is a very popular sweetener; chewable tablets can contain more than 50% and liquid formulation may contain up to 85% sucrose. Its ubiquity is due to the combination of sweetness and functional properties (highly soluble, viscosity enhancer, preservative at high concentration, texture enhancer) and high-intensity sweetness. Sucrose is broken down in the stomach by acidic hydrolysis into its component sugars, which are then absorbed into the bloodstream through the intestine. It has been linked with some adverse health effects. The most common is tooth decay, in which bacteria in the mouth convert sucrose to produce acids that attack tooth enamel.

Table 4.4 Relative sweetness to sucrose of various sweeteners

Sweetener	Relative sweetness
Sucrose	1
Lactose	0.4
Mannitol	0.5–0.7
Sorbitol	0.6
Glycerol	0.6
Glucose	0.7
Maltitol	0.9
Xylitol	1
Fructose	1.4
Cyclamate	30–50
Acesulfame potassium	100–200
Aspartame	180–200
Sodium saccharin	250–500
Neohesperidin dihydrochalcone	340
Sucralose	500–600
Thaumatin	2000–3000
Neotame	8000–13 000

Sucrose has high food energy content (4 cal/g or 17 kJ/g) and in a poorly managed diet can contribute to obesity. This is a dose-dependent side effect and children with diabetes mellitus need to control their intake of sucrose along with the other carbohydrates. Rinsing the mouth after taking a formulation containing sucrose is recommended, especially after intake of viscous formulations that may have a prolonged contact time in the oral cavity. This could help to overcome the cariogenic effect as it takes about 24 hours for a large enough build-up of bacteria to accumulate on a tooth to produce cavity-causing acid (Bigeard, 2000).

The older name of glucose is 'dextrose' – because a solution of D-glucose rotates polarised light towards the right. In the same vein D-fructose was called 'laevulose' because a solution of levulose rotates polarised light to the left. Despite having the sweetest taste of all natural sugars, fructose (corn syrup) is not widely used in formulation. Compared with glucose, its hepatic metabolism favours lipogenesis, which may contribute to hyperlipidaemia and obesity, but fructose does not increase insulin levels (Havel, 2005). The term 'invert sugar' describes an equimolar mix of glucose and fructose.

Lactose is a disaccharide consisting of two subunits, a galactose and a glucose, but is the least sweet of the natural sugars. There is a fairly high occurrence of lactose intolerance in adulthood. It is the condition in which lactase, an enteric brush border enzyme needed for proper metabolism of lactose (a constituent of milk and other dairy products), is not present. Not commonly used in liquids, lactose is widely used as a filler or diluent in tablets and capsules and to give bulk to powders. Sensitivity to lactose varies widely in severity, although some adults and children may experience diarrhoea, gaseousness or cramping after ingestion of as little as 3 g lactose and possibly less. In some patients, 100–200 mg can cause intestinal disorders (Gundend-However *et al.*, 1970).

Similarly, povidone, a common pharmaceutical polymer used as a viscosity enhancer, a suspending, stabilising agent in liquids and a wet or dry binder and disintegrant in solid dosage forms, has been shown to be responsible for an anaphylactic reaction (Pedrosa *et al.*, 2005).

Sugar alcohols or polyols are commercially produced from glucose, or derived from fruit and vegetables. The most common sugar alcohols are sorbitol, mannitol, maltitol and xylitol. Sugar alcohols are recognised as not contributing to tooth decay or causing increases in blood glucose. They are absorbed more slowly than conventional sugars, thus they do not contribute to a rapid rise in blood sugar level and the resultant insulin response. This may be the reason why they can have an osmotic laxative effect that can reduce bioavailability of some drugs (e.g. Biopharmaceutics Classification System [BCS] class III drugs). These sugar alcohols are called a nutritive sweetener because they provide fewer calories (about 40%) than sugars with an equivalent sweetness. Ingesting large amounts of polyols can lead to some abdominal pain, flatulence and mild- to severe-diarrhoea. Sorbitol is often used. It is metabolised to fructose and is therefore unsuitable for people intolerant to fructose. Mannitol has a tendency to lose a hydrogen ion in aqueous solutions, which causes the solution to become acidic. It is therefore not uncommon to add a buffer to maintain its pH. Mannitol also has a negative heat of solution. For this reason, mannitol is used as a sweetener in chewing tablets, the cooling effect adding to the fresh feel. This effect can also be used to mask bitter tastes. Glycerol is also often used in formulations but its sweetening power is weaker. Mannitol and glycerol can be administered intravenously.

Artificial sweeteners can be used in conjunction with sugars and polyols to enhance the degree of sweetness, or on their own in formulations to restrict the sugar intake. Artificial sweeteners have the disadvantage of imparting a slightly bitter and metallic aftertaste. Sodium cyclamate is the least potent of the commercially used artificial sweeteners. Some patients find that it has an unpleasant aftertaste, but generally less so than saccharin or acesulfame potassium. It is often used synergistically with other artificial sweeteners, especially saccharin; the mixture of 10 parts cyclamate to 1 part saccharin is common and masks the off-tastes of both sweeteners. It is less expensive than most sweeteners, including sucrose, and is stable under heat. In the 1960s, a study reported that some intestinal bacteria could desulfonate cyclamate to produce cyclohexylamine, a compound suspected to have some chronic toxicity in animals. Further research found the common 10:1 cyclamate:saccharin mixture to increase the incidence of bladder cancer in rats. It is banned for pharmaceutical use in the USA and Canada but its use is restricted only in some countries in Europe (E950).

Acesulfame potassium is heat stable under moderately acidic or basic conditions but unstable at low pH. It is approved for safety everywhere and is often blended with other sweeteners. These blends are reputed to give a more sugar-like taste where each sweetener masks the other's aftertaste, and to exhibit a synergistic effect wherein the blend is sweeter than its components.

Aspartame is the methyl ester of two amino acids: aspartic acid and phenylalanine. Aspartame provides the same energy as any protein,

4 cal/g, but this is not significant due to the small amount needed to sweeten products. Due to a possible excess of phenylalanine in children with phenylketonuria, aspartame must carry a warning label. Phenylketonuria is a genetic disease in which the body cannot produce the enzyme necessary to use phenylalanine; symptoms are headache and nervousness. Many commercial products contain aspartame (e.g. NutraSweet). The use of aspartame is limited at high or prolonged temperatures and in solution because it breaks down and loses its sweetness; it may also produce toxic metabolites (methanol) and in rare cases individuals may have a sensitivity to aspartame.

Saccharin sodium is the oldest artificial sweetener. It is a sulfanilamide derivative and is stable within a wide range of temperatures but, in the presence of acids, does react chemically, and therefore is not compatible with preservatives that require low pH. In its acidic form, saccharin is not particularly water soluble. Therefore, the form used is usually the sodium salt. The calcium salt is also sometimes used, especially for restricting dietary sodium intake. Many studies have been carried out on saccharin, with some showing a correlation between saccharin consumption and increased cancer (especially bladder cancer) and others showing no such correlation. Nevertheless, no study has ever shown health risks in humans when saccharin is taken at normal doses. It has been approved for use in the USA but not in Canada, and was approved for use in Europe for children over 3 years of age.

Neohesperidin dihydrochalcone, sometimes abbreviated to neohesperidin DC or simply NHDC, is an artificial sweetener derived from citrus fruit. Its potency is naturally affected by such factors as the application for which it is used and the pH of the product. Like other highly sweet glycosides, such as glycyrrhizin (from the liquorice root) and those found in stevia, NHDC's sweet taste has a slower onset than sugars and lingers in the mouth for some time. Unlike aspartame, NHDC remains stable at elevated temperatures and in acidic or basic conditions, and so can be used in applications that require a long shelf-life. The EU has approved NHDC's use (E959) but it has not been approved as a sweetener in the USA, although it is considered a generally recognised as safe (GRAS) 'flavour enhancer'.

NHDC is well known for having a strong synergistic effect when used in conjunction with other artificial sweeteners such as aspartame, saccharin and acesulfame potassium, as well as sugar alcohols such as xylitol and cyclamate. NHDC usage boosts the effects of these sweeteners at lower concentrations than would otherwise be required; smaller amounts of other sweeteners are needed. This provides a cost benefit.

It is noted particularly for enhancing sensory effects ('mouth feel') and can be used as a means of reducing the bitterness of pharmacological drugs. It is used as an artificial sweetener at around 15–20 parts per million (ppm). Research has shown that, at strengths of around and above 20 ppm, NHDC can produce side effects such as nausea and migraine.

Sucralose (Splenda) is manufactured by the selective chlorination of sucrose, in which three of sucrose's hydroxyl groups are substituted with chlorine atoms. Unlike aspartame, it is stable under heat and over a broad pH range. It has a pleasant, long-lasting, sweet taste similar to sucrose, in contrast with other intensive sweeteners. It was initially believed that sucralose was entirely excreted. Because chlorinated compounds (such as DDT and other pesticides) may be stored in body fat, the belief that it was not absorbed diminished health concerns initially. But the US Food and Drug Administation (FDA) determined that up to about 27% of sucralose can be absorbed by the body, igniting concern over the dangers of elevated chlorine levels in the body. Ironically, bonded chlorine is found in common foods, such as table salt, and it is excreted by the body. However, the chlorine in sucralose forms a covalent bond with carbon and does not form the chloride ions that can be renally excreted. Sucralose has withstood the scrutiny of several national and international food safety regulatory bodies with the exception of Japan.

Highly water-soluble thaumatin is a mixture of intensely sweet proteins (thaumatins) extracted with water from the arils of the fruit of the West African perennial plant *Thaumatococcus daniellii*. The thaumatins have a normal complement of amino acids, except that histidine is not present. Extensive disulfide cross-linking confers thermal stability, resistance to denaturation (e.g. heating under acidic conditions) and maintenance of the tertiary structure of the polypeptide chain, which is critical to thaumatin's technical function. Cleavage of just one disulfide bridge results in a loss of sweet taste. Thaumatin has been approved as a sweetener in the EU, Israel and Japan. In the USA, it is a GRAS flavouring agent, but since 2005 it is not approved as a sweetener. Safety data is unproven in children.

Neotame is an artificial sweetener derived from and similar in structure to aspartame. However, neotame is heat stable, much more potent and of no danger to those suffering from phenylketonuria, as it is not metabolised into phenylalanine. Peptidases, which would typically break the peptide bond between the aspartic acid and phenylalanine moieties, are essentially blocked by the presence of the

3,3-dimethylbutyl moiety. Neotame is rapidly metabolised, completely eliminated and does not accumulate in the body. It is GRAS listed and approved as a food in many countries.

Flavouring and colouring agents

There are many taste-masking strategies. Using flavouring agents is one strategy to make medicines more acceptable, especially if the drug has an unpleasant taste, despite the use of a sweetening agent. They can be either natural (natural flavours extracted from fruit or vegetables or essential oils extracted from plant fractions) or artificial. 'Nature-identical' flavours are the chemical equivalent of natural flavours, just chemically synthesised rather than being extracted from the original source. Obviously, if flavouring agents contain alcohol they will not be the preferred choice for paediatric products.

Many of the compounds used to produce artificial flavour belong to the chemical category of esters. The list of known flavouring agents includes hundreds of molecular compounds, and they are often mixed together to produce many of the common flavours.

While there are many studies on the toxicity of colouring agents, there are very few on pharmaceutical flavouring agents. Nevertheless, a variety of allergic or pseudo-allergic reactions have been described, such as hypersentivity reactions, systemic allergic reactions and respiratory depression, as with menthol, for example.

Natural or synthetic colouring agents or dyes can be added to match the taste (e.g. yellow for a banana taste) in order to improve the attractiveness of the product or, more appropriately in children, to enable easy product identification, particularly in the case of poisonous materials (e.g. green methadone mixture, external antiseptic). Colouring agents or dyes can also be used to mask an unpleasant drug colour or coloured degradation products, which do not always affect the use of the preparation but can hinder an easy visual appreciation of the quality of the preparation.

In pharmacy, the dyes used are azo dyes, quinoline dyes, triphenylmethane and xanthine dyes. They are not recommended in children because many colouring agents, mainly synthetic dyes, have been associated with hypersensitivity and other adverse reactions (gastrointestinal intolerance, dermatological reactions and carcinogenic concerns). Approximately 2–20% of people with asthma are sensitive to aspirin. Cross-reactions to azo dyes such as tartrazine produce similar effects. They have occurred in patients both with and without a history of aspirin intolerance, and include acute bronchospasm, non-immuno-logical urticaria, eosinophilia and angioedema. Patients with the classic aspirin triad reaction (asthma, urticaria and rhinitis) or non-immuno-logical anaphylactoid reactions may develop similar reactions to dyes such as tartrazine, amaranth, erythrosine, indigo carmine, ponceau, new coccine, sunset yellow, brilliant blue, methyl blue and quinolone yellow (American Academy for Pediatrics: Committee on Drugs, 1997). Natural dyes are generally considered to be weaker sensitisers.

Preservatives

A preservative is a natural or more often a synthetic chemical added to pharmaceutical products to retard spoilage, whether from microbial growth or undesirable chemical changes. Antimicrobial preservatives function by inhibiting the growth of bacteria and fungi, and antioxidants inhibit the oxidation process within the preparation. They can be incorporated in various preparations intended for use via various routes of administration. As an example of the variety of preservatives used, Table 4.5 lists the preservatives being used within the London region NHS pharmaceutical manufacturing units as of May 2004 (Rabiu *et al.*, 2004).

Antimicrobial preservatives are generally added to liquid preparations to prevent or reduce microbial growth. Despite being banned in the USA since 1976 and in many other countries, chloroform is still in use to preserve oral medication. It is limited in the UK to a content of 0.5% (w/w or w/v) but usually used at 0.25%. Chloroform should be considered an obsolete preservative for pharmaceutical preparations, especially paediatric preparations, because of its toxicological and carcinogenic implications and its volatility. Benzoic acid, sodium benzoate and benzyl alcohol (which is metabolised to benzoic acid) are aromatic alcohols used in a wide variety of formulations as preservatives. Benzoic acid has been implicated as the agent responsible for precipitating 'gasping syndrome' in premature neonates. Ethanol and propylene glycol are also used to a varying extent and their toxicities have been discussed already. The term 'parabens' refers to a suitable combination of methyl parahydroxybenzoate and propyl parahydroxybenzoate at a final concentration of 0.1% w/v. They are generally safe although should be avoided as much as possible in critically ill neonates with jaundice, kernicterus and hyperbilirubinaemia, because their metabolism and excretion pathways could cause displacement of bilirubin from albumin and accumulation in the body. Use of benzalkonium

Table 4.5 Preservatives being used within the London region NHS pharmaceutical manufacturing units as of May 2004

Preservatives	Uses			
	Internal medication	Sterile preparation	External medication	Extemporaneous preparation
Chloroform	✓			✓
Benzoic acid	✓			
Ethanol	✓			
Propylene glycol	✓		✓	✓
Potassium sorbate	✓			
Methyl parabens	✓			✓
Sodium methyl parabens	✓			✓
Propyl parabens	✓			✓
Benzyl alcohol			✓	✓
Benzalkonium chloride[a]		✓		
Chlorhexidine[a]		✓		
Phenyl mercuric nitrate[a]		✓		
Thiomersal[a]		✓		

[a]Ophthalmic preparation.
Reproduced with permission from Rabiu *et al.* (2004).

chloride is not recommended, especially in anti-asthma products, as it has been reported to have side effects on the respiratory tract. Chlorbutanol is mainly used in ophthalmic and parenteral preparation. It is a mild sedative and analgesic which has incompatibilities with other excipients. It is not recommended internally.

Antioxidant preservatives added to oral preparations are commonly ascorbic acid, citric acid and sodium metabisulfites. They are odourless and tasteless, and supposed to be non-toxic. Nevertheless, sulfites have been incriminated in allergic-type reactions, including anaphylaxis, by many routes of administration.

Labelling should state clearly the excipient composition of the medicine so that predictable harmful effects can be avoided, especially in very young patients. For the formulator, the choice of excipients should be guided by a thorough risk assessment of the excipients, the route of administration and the patient susceptibility. It is highly recommended to refer to manuals such as authorities' guidelines, pharmacopoeias, a handbook of excipients and the latest literature available.

Paediatric drug delivery and routes of administration

By definition, drug delivery systems allow patients to take their medication in a convenient and effective manner. They are designed to be the most appropriate dosage form to suit the patient and to treat a specific disease. Ultimately, efficacy and safety while limiting side effects are improved along with compliance.

The potential of various routes of administration in children will be addressed briefly, bearing in mind that, when choosing a route in a defined clinical situation, the same general rules apply as in adult administration. Nevertheless, this choice will also be influenced by the developmental stage of the child and is further complicated by the capability and cooperation of the children and their carers.

Oral and rectal routes

Oral route

Administration of any medicine per os remains the route of choice if the clinical condition allows it.

Liquid oral medicines have the advantage of dose versatility and ease of administration even through nasogastric tubes. They are limited by the volume possible or practical to administer, acute taste, possible inaccuracy or loss at administration, restricted choice and levels of suitable excipients, stability issues and the lack of modified release. The dosing device (dropper, measuring spoon, graduated pipette, oral syringe) becomes extremely important, especially for accurately measuring small volumes of a narrow therapeutic index drug (e.g. phenytoin).

Monolithic solid dosage form can avoid palatability issues if swallowed intact, but, depending on their age and training, many children are unable to swallow whole tablets or capsules (Czyzewski et al., 2000). Evidence of preference and acceptability has to be further investigated as few anecdotal studies on this issue have been carried out. With solid dosage forms, stability is improved and modified release can be achieved, but the lack of dose flexibility can be a drawback. The use of mini-platforms, such as mini-tablets, mini-capsules or spheroids with an appropriate dispensing system, could overcome this problem. Nevertheless, age-related ability and safety (aspiration, choking) when taking these medicines should be taken into consideration and investigated.

Effervescent preparations, powders and granules, chewable dosage forms and fast-dissolving/disintegrating preparations in the oral cavity, such as tablets or strips/films/wafers, stand on the periphery of solids and liquids. They all have the advantages of solids in that they are compact and more stable but they also have the same palatability issues as liquids, with the particular challenge that the quantity of excipients available to improve the taste is limited. Literature suggests that chewable tablets provide a safe, well-tolerated alternative in children over 2 years of age who have teeth (Michele *et al.*, 2002). Unlike fast-dissolving/disintegrating tablets (FDDTs) and films, they can be spat out easily and, unlike effervescent preparations, powders and granules but like FDDTs, they do not require food or drink for administration.

Buccal and sublingual routes

For local but also systemic delivery, the oromucosal route might be suitable if safety is established. Mucoadhesive preparations, especially films, semi-solids and liquids, might be of interest if they do not inter-fere with suction and frequent feeding. Nevertheless, one of the major issues remains the taste of the preparation and the willingness as well as the ability of the child to retain buccal or sublingual tablets in the mouth, thus ensuring that sufficient absorption takes place.

Rectal route

Rectal administration of solids is not dose flexible and absorption is poorly reproducible. It is affected by active non-compliance (poorly accepted by older children or caregivers) or passive non-compliance (premature ejection when it should be retained for at least 20/30 minutes). Lubricants are sometimes used to ease insertion, although it is unclear whether the release and absorption of the drug are modified when using this method. Water could be a valuable lubricant. If the appropriate size/dose of suppository is not available, as illustrated in Figure 4.4, splitting the suppository is not recommended (see under Solid dosage forms, page 47).

Other semi-liquid or liquid preparations can be used rectally (gel, enemas). Rectal drug delivery should not be overlooked in certain thera-peutic situations, when oral and parenteral routes are not available, or when the child is unconscious (e.g. postoperative), vomiting or on continuous suction. The absorption is usually rapid and may avoid first-pass metabolism.

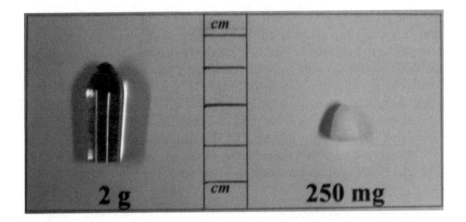

Figure 4.4 Paediatric suppositories.

Ocular and aural routes

Ear and eye routes of administration are never well tolerated, especially by children, but are very often unavoidable when treating topical conditions. Moreover, it is difficult to administer the treatment in an optimised way as it requires dexterity of the carer and a high level of cooperation from the patient, which might be difficult to achieve in younger children. Prolonged-release preparations that would decrease the frequency of administration might be better accepted and improve the efficacy of these topical treatments.

Dermal and transdermal routes

Adequately formulated topical delivery to treat disorders of the skin is generally well tolerated. Nevertheless, any possible toxic effects must be eradicated, especially as percutaneous passage during childhood can be greater, particularly in younger children (up to 2 years old).

Occlusion of semi-solid preparations may be useful if systemic absorption is desired. A careful risk–benefit evaluation is then required. Transdermal patches are a more elegant alternative. Being virtually painless and easy to apply, if they achieve controlled delivery, they provide a formulation of choice for prolonged-release systemic uptake. They would have to be adapted to skin maturation, formulated with adhesives with low allergenic potential and be available in different strengths. Of course, the same inter- and intra-patient variability in relation to sites of administration and skin condition occurs in children as in adults.

Respiratory routes

Nasal administration is also intended mainly for local effects (ointments, drops or sprays) but it can provide direct access to the systemic circulation. The development of mechanical dispensing systems adapted for dose volume and the dimensions of the patient's nose may prove a valuable alternative to invasive modes of systemic administration, mainly through the respiratory region of the nose. Strong possibilities are peptides (e.g. desmopressin), vaccines, as they are administered as early as neonatal age, and emergency drugs (e.g. opiates for acute severe pain) and for drugs to be delivered through the olfactory region to the blood–brain barrier. Absorption is comparable to intravenous administration.

Asthma is prevalent during childhood. The pulmonary route is well established, although self-administration is difficult for younger patients. The choice of inhalation devices is crucial and is made in relation to age. Guidelines on the following are available on the National Institute for Health and Clinical Excellence (NICE) website (2005a,b):

- Both corticosteroids and bronchodilator therapy should routinely be delivered by a pressurised metered dose inhaler (pMDI) and spacer system, with a facemask where necessary in infants, toddlers and children under 5 years of age.
- Where this combination is not clinically effective for the child and, depending on the child's condition, nebulised therapy may be considered. In the case of children aged 3–5, a dry powder inhaler (DPI) may also be considered but usually DPIs are used in school-age children (>5 years old).
- The choice of which pMDI device and spacer to use should be determined by the specific needs of the child and the likelihood of compliance.

Many years ago, the USA agreed with other countries to stop using CFCs (chlorofluorocarbons) as propellants in aerosols because they contribute to the destruction of the atmospheric ozone layer. Until recently, formulary exemptions were made for inhalers that contained CFCs. The pMDI remains the most popular type of inhaler used by people with asthma, with a different propellant called hydrofluoroalkane (HFA), also referred to as CFC-free propellant. It may be less powerful and have a different taste which could impair compliance and efficacy in children accustomed to using their old inhaler. The DPI is the second most popular type of inhaler; it uses the patient's inspiratory flow to deliver the powdered drug to the lungs. DPIs might be easier for children with sufficient inspiratory flow rate as they do not require coordination between actuation and inspiration. Although the pulmonary route is mainly used for local therapy, it might become more important in the future for systemic delivery of drugs such as insulin or other labile drugs per os.

Parenteral routes

In hospital, many patients have a venous cannula and systemic drugs not given orally are usually given intravenously (i.v.) rather than subcutaneously (s.c.) or intramuscularly (i.m.). Other parenteral routes of administration (intrathecal, epidural, intra-osseous, subcutaneous infusion, intra-arterial, intracardiac, etc.) can be used by trained staff but they are restricted to marginal use (e.g. palliative care, emergency situations such as resuscitation). Parenteral routes allow the administration of drugs to unconscious, uncooperative, dehydrated patients and for chemotherapy. Drugs that are inactive or irritable via other routes can also be administered via this route. The dose administered is complete and accurate. There is a fast onset of therapeutic action as the systemic effect is direct, with predictable bioavailability. There is no first-pass metabolism. Nevertheless, once administered, the effect cannot be reversed (e.g. in case of overdose).

Administration usually creates pain, anxiety and phobia, and requires professionally trained staff. Topical anaesthesia (creams, gels, patches or simply cold to numb the area) is usually performed to help to manage the pain and associated fears, as well as to distract the child. There is no taste issue with the parenteral routes but the excipients used must be biodegradable under the available metabolic processes. This can be a problem in neonates as not all pathways have fully matured. Moreover, formulation composition is critical as some excipients can be toxic. This includes vehicles, preservatives or even the antiseptic used to disinfect the surface of the skin prior to injection (e.g. iodine-containing antiseptic that can be absorbed through the skin).

The cost of parenteral administration can be high due to the need for frequent dosing and the requirement for aseptic/sterile conditions for preparation of the doses. Moreover, dosing errors due to calculation and/or dilution errors are not uncommon, especially in neonates and infants, as they require frequent dose adaptation, serial dilutions to achieve measurable volumes or withdrawal of a dose volume that is less

Table 4.6 Fluid and sodium requirements per 24 hours

Requirements	Per 24 hours	Comment
Body weight		
<3 kg	150 mL/kg	Start at 40–60 mL/kg if newborn
3–10 kg	100 mL/kg	Maximum 2000 mL in woman and 2500 mL in man
For each kilogram between 10 and 20 kg	Add 50 mL/kg	
For each kilogram >20 kg	Add 20 mL/kg	
Sodium	3 mmol/kg	

Adapted from Royal College of Paediatrics and Child Health and Neonatal Paediatric Pharmacists Group (2003) with permission from RCPCH Publications Ltd.

than the total volume in the vial. The volume of the injection has to be considered in relation to the fluid and sodium requirements of children of various ages and weights (Table 4.6). Those requirements include treatment and nutritional fluids. Appropriate compatible dilution fluids, such as glucose 5 or 10% and sodium chloride 0.45 or 0.9%, have to be used.

Many hospital pharmacies provide doses of certain intravenously administered drugs as ready-to-use injections in syringes or small-volume infusions. These are prepared aseptically at the Centralised Intravenous Additive Service (CIVAS). The stability of further diluted commercial preparations has to be established, if not stated by the manufacturer.

The intravenous route is used to deliver larger volumes (e.g. replacement and hyperalimentation solutions). Positioning catheters in a central vein's blood flow avoids multiple injections in seriously ill patients. Rapid dilution occurs compared to injection in peripheral veins. In the latter, infiltration, phlebitis due to osmolarity, pH and the characteristic of the drug and excipients can damage the vessels and lead to the loss of veins for therapy. Other common risks encountered with intravenous administration include activity restriction, impact of normal fluctuations in feeding, activity and sleeping patterns, the pulling out of intravenous lines by the patient, infection and extravasion.

Subcutaneously, small volumes (<2 mL) should be used to avoid pain. The size of the needle (short and high gauge number) should be chosen in proportion to the child. Automatic needle insertion appears to be less painful and to improve compliance in the long term (e.g. insulin therapy). The preferred sites of injection are the upper arm, lower abdomen and anterior and lateral thighs, and injection sites should be rotated to avoid lipodystrophy and other tissue formations. A few formulation tricks can alleviate pain at injection; the pH should be physiological, for example. Citrate-free and low ionic strength preparations can also help. Usually, isotonic solutions are given.

In premature infants, inefficient muscle contractions and vasomotor activity affect drug absorption. Therefore, pharmacokinetic characteristics after an intramuscular injection can be altered and difficult to predict. The intramuscular route is very painful in younger children but the pain can be eased by choosing the most appropriate size of needle (longer and with lower gauge number), by administering small volumes and by choosing the right site of injection: generally in the thigh, in the upper outer quadrant of the buttock for older children or in the deltoid muscle, which tends to be underdeveloped in younger patients. Common adverse effects can be muscle contraction and nerve injury, as well as abscess formation. Intramuscular injections should be avoided in children with coagulation defects. The intramuscular route should be used only to administer a one-off dose if other routes of administration are unusable.

More investigation is needed into transcutaneous delivery. Needle-free systems such as 'jet injectors', which force liquid or powdered drug though the skin by the means of compressed gas, could be an alternative if discomfort (bruising) is minimised. The microneedle system of delivery also seems very promising. Compared with hypodermic needles, microneedles do not significantly stimulate nerve endings and are thus well tolerated.

Administration of medications to children can be stressful, traumatic and sub-therapeutic if the formulation is unsuitable. Finding an ideal delivery system for children is a real challenge; it should be: accurate; suit all age groups; have a minimal dosage frequency; have good palatability; contain few, non-toxic excipients; be easy for the child to take or for the carer to administer; and be a robust and stable formulation and commercially viable. As awareness of the importance of preparing tailored medicines for children increases, knowledge of paediatric drug delivery is expected to grow dramatically in the near future, thus increasing the availability of better medicines.

References

American Academy for Pediatrics: Committee on Drugs (1997). 'Inactive' ingredients in pharmaceutical products: Update (Subject Review). *Pediatrics* 99: 268–278.

Bigeard L (2000). The role of medication and sugars in pediatric dental patients. *Pediatr Dent* 44: 443–456.

Breitkreutz J, Wessel T, Boos J (1999). Dosage forms for peroral drug administration to children. *Paediatr Perinat Drug Ther* 3: 25–33.

Czyzewski D I, Runyan D R, Lopez M A, *et al.* (2000). Teaching and maintaining pill swallowing in HIV-infected children. *AIDS Read* 10: 88–94.

European Commission (2006). Medicines for Children. http://pharmacos.eudra.org/F2/Paediatrics/index.htm (accessed 19 October 2006).

Gundend-However E, Dahlquist A, Jarnum S (1970). The clinical significance of lactose malabsorption. *Am J Gastroenterol* 53: 460–471.

Havel P J (2005). Dietary fructose: implications for dysregulation of energy homeostasis and lipid/carbohydrate metabolism. *Nutr Rev* 63: 133–157.

Hofer K N, McCarthy M W, Buck M L, *et al.* (2003). Possible anaphylaxis after propofol in a child with food allergy. *Ann Pharmacother* 37: 398–401.

Michele T M, Knorr B, Vadas E B, Reiss T F (2002). Safety of chewable tablets for children. *J Asthma* 39: 391–403.

Nahata M C, Hipple T F (2003). *Pediatric Drug Formulations*, 5th edn. Cincinnati, OH: Harvey Whitney Books Co.

National Institute for Health and Clinical Excellence (2005a). Technology Appraisal Guidance no. 10, on inhaler systems (devices) in children under the age of 5 years with chronic asthma. http://www.nice.org.uk/page.aspx?o=TA10 (accessed 19 October 2006).

National Institute for Health and Clinical Excellence (2005b). Technology Appraisal Guidance no. 38, on inhaler devices for routine treatment of chronic asthma in older children (aged 5–15 years) http://www.nice.org.uk/page.aspx?o=TA38 (accessed 19 October 2006).

Paddock Laboratories Inc. (2003). Compounding Bibliography: List of over 60 published extemporaneously oral liquid stability studies. http://www.paddocklabs.com/biblog_working.html#top (accessed 19 October 2006).

Pedrosa C, Costa H, Oliveira G, *et al.* (2005). Anaphylaxis to povidone in a child. *Pediatr Allergy Immunol* 16: 361–362.

Rabiu F, Forsey P, Patel S (2004). Preservatives can produce harmful effects in paediatric drug preparations. *Pharm Pract* May: 101–108.

Royal College of Paediatrics and Child Health and Neonatal Paediatric Pharmacists Group (2003). Intravenous fluid therapy. In: *Medicines for Children*, 2nd edn. London: RCPCH Publications, G54–57.

Savolainen H (2005). Propylene glycol toxicity. *Chest eLetters*, http://www.chestjournal.org/cgi/eletters/128/3/1674 (accessed 19 October 2006).

Standing J, Tuleu C (2005). Paediatric formulation – getting to the heart of the problem. *Int J Pharm* 300: 56–66.

Teng J, Song C K, Williams R L, *et al.* (2002). Lack of medication dose uniformity in commonly split tablets. *J Am Pharm Assoc* 42: 195–199.

Tuleu C, Grangé J, Seurin S (2005). The need of paediatric formulation: administration of nifedipine in children, a proof of concept. *J Drug Del Sci Tech* 15: 319–324.

Yeung V, Tuleu C, Wong I (2004). Extemporaneous manipulation of drugs in a paediatric hospital pharmacy: a national audit. *Paediatr Perinatal Drug Ther* 6: 75–80.

Wilson K, Reardon C, Theodore A C, *et al.* (2005) Propylene glycol toxicity: a severe iatrogenic illness in ICU patients receiving IV benzodiazepines: a case series and prospective, observational pilot study. *Chest* 128: 1674–1681.

Wong I C K, Ghaleb M, Dean Franklin B, *et al.* (2004). Incidence and nature of dosing errors in paediatric medications – a systematic review. *Drug Safety* 27: 661–670.

Woods D J (2001). *Formulation in Pharmacy Practice*, 2nd edn. Pharminfotech (CD-ROM).

5

Updates and regulations around the world

Ian K Wong

Introduction

The regulations and initiatives related to the research and development of children's medicines have been rapidly changing in the USA and European Union (EU) since the 1990s. The USA is taking the lead in reforming the regulatory system in order to improve research into children's medicines and increase the availability of licensed medicines for children. The EU is closely following the lead of the USA and new regulations and various research initiatives have already started. In this chapter, you will be introduced to various initiatives in the USA and EU.

Regulatory changes in the USA

Final Rule

In 1979, a 'paediatric use' sub-section was introduced to the product information (PI), which was intended to inspire paediatric medicines research. Unfortunately, this did not materialise. The US Food and Drug Administration (FDA) then proposed a new regulation in 1992 designed to improve information on paediatric drugs supplied for approval. The regulation was approved in 1994 (the Final Rule) (Food and Drug Administration, 1994). The Final Rule required pharmaceutical manufacturers to re-examine existing data to determine whether those data could be modified to include paediatric use information on the basis of adult studies and available paediatric data.

If the existing data allowed adaptation of the paediatric use information, a supplemental new drug application was required to be submitted to the FDA for approval of a change in the PI. In this situation if there was insufficient information to support use of the drug in children, manufacturers were required to include a statement in the PI regarding the limitations (e.g. 'Safety and effectiveness in paediatric patients below certain age have not been established'). However, the Final Rule did not place constraints on manufacturers to conduct the necessary studies in the absence of inadequate existing data. Despite the potential for the medicines to be used in children, manufacturers were allowed to place a disclaimer in the PI rather than conducting the necessary studies. As a result, the Final Rule did not have significant effects on children's medicines research.

Pediatric Rule

In 1997 the Pediatric Rule (Food and Drug Administration, 1998) was proposed. This required manufacturers of most new and marketed drugs to conduct studies to provide adequate paediatric drug information. The Pediatric Rule is a much more regulatory approach to paediatric labelling. These regulations establish the presumption that all not-yet-approved new drugs and biological products must be studied in paediatric patients, and assert the authority to require paediatric studies for currently marketed new drugs and biologics. However, manufacturers may obtain waivers from the paediatric studies' requirement if the product (1) does not represent a meaningful therapeutic benefit over existing treatments for children and (2) is not likely to be used in a substantial number of children.

For currently marketed drugs and biological products, the rule authorises the FDA to require paediatric studies if (1) they are used for a labelled indication in a substantial number of children (defined as 50 000 or more) and the absence of adequate labelling could pose a significant risk to children, or (2) the product would provide a meaningful therapeutic benefit over existing treatments of children and the absence of labelling could impose significant risks. Waivers are available for marketed drugs if (1) paediatric studies are impossible or highly impractical (e.g. the patient populations are small or geographically diverse) or (2) evidence suggests strongly that the product would be ineffective or unsafe in children.

Food and Drug Administration Modernisation Act

The Pediatric Rule was finalised in 1998 and became effective on 1 April 1999. After the proposed Pediatric Rule was issued but before it was finalised, the Food and Drug Administration Modernisation Act (FDAMA) (Food and Drug Administration, 1997) was enacted by the

US Senate and House of Representatives. Also called the Paediatric Exclusivity Provision, the House of Representatives set up economic incentives for manufacturers who voluntarily conducted studies in children for new medicines or medicines that were on a prioritised list drawn up by the US Secretary of Health and Human Services. A 6-month extension to existing exclusive or listed patent protection was given to selected new and already marketed drugs for which paediatric use data had been submitted. In 2001, a report to Congress regarding the FDAMA stated that the 'Paediatric Exclusivity Provision has done more to generate clinical studies and useful prescribing information for the paediatric population than any other regulatory or legislative process to date' (Department of Health and Human Services, 2001). In the 2 years following this legislative change there were over five times the number of paediatric studies completed compared with the preceding 5 years.

However, despite the FDAMA's success in increasing the number of medicines with paediatric drug use information, there were concerns that the medicines being studied may not be of greatest need in children but medicines with the greatest potential for financial gain. Further problems with the FDAMA were also apparent: patent extension under the FDAMA could be granted only to medicines with market exclusivity or still under patent protection. Patent extension was an inadequate incentive for drugs with low sales, since there would not be a large enough market return to compensate for the cost of conducting paediatric studies. The FDAMA was also unable to encourage the production of data in younger age groups (e.g. neonates), for whom an appropriate clinical trial could not be designed until studies in older children had been submitted and analysed. Once paediatric exclusivity was granted for studies in the older age groups, there were insufficient incentives to enable later studies in the younger age groups. Additionally, there was a very limited subset of medicines in which a second period of exclusivity was applicable.

Best Pharmaceuticals for Children Act

The enactment by Congress of the Best Pharmaceuticals for Children Act (BPCA) (Food and Drug Administration, 2002) in 2002 led to the re-authorisation of the paediatric exclusivity incentive programme under the FDAMA. The BPCA not only renewed the exclusivity provision under the FDAMA, but also established an additional mechanism for obtaining paediatric drug information for off-patent medicines. Under the BPCA, the National Institutes of Health (equivalent to the Medical Research Council in the UK) provide public funding to conduct research on those medicines that manufacturers opted not to test in children.

The BPCA also established an Office of Paediatric Therapeutics within the FDA to oversee and coordinate paediatric activities and programmes, and the reporting of all adverse events for one year after exclusivity has been granted. Furthermore, the results of completed paediatric studies must be made public.

Pediatric Research Equity Act

In October 2002 the Washington DC Federal District Court overturned the Pediatric Rule. The court pointed out that the US Congress never intended the FDA to have the statutory authority to require paediatric drug studies. In 2003, the Pediatric Research Equity Act (PREA) was enacted (Food and Drug Administration, 2003). The PREA stipulated that all applications for new active ingredients, indication, dosage form, dosing regimen or route of administration must contain a paediatric assessment unless a deferral or waiver of paediatric studies has been obtained. The paediatric assessment must contain data adequate to assess a drug's safety and effectiveness, including dosing regimens in children. Deferrals may be granted in situations where a drug is ready for approval for use in adults before paediatric studies are complete or paediatric studies should be delayed until additional safety or effectiveness data are made available. Waivers from a paediatric assessment may be applied (see section above). In the case of a waiver, the PREA could require manufacturers to include in the PI a statement indicating that waivers from a paediatric assessment have been granted because the drug was found to be ineffective or unsafe for children. The PREA has the sunset date of 10 January 2007.

Network of paediatric pharmacology research units in the USA

The most commonly cited reasons for lack of research into paediatric medicines are (Wong et al., 2003):

1. High cost compared with potential return
2. Complex ethical issues including consent, accents and the use of placebo

3.   Too few qualified paediatric pharmacology investigators to plan and conduct studies.

In order to tackle problems 2 and 3, the US National Institute of Child Health and Human Development (NICHD) provided funding to establish a network of paediatric pharmacology research units (PPRUs) (Paediatric Pharmacology Research Unit Network, 2006) in 1994. The mission of the PPRUs is to facilitate and promote paediatric labelling of new drugs or drugs already on the market, and the Network provided a ready source of trained, experienced and skilled clinical investigators. There are currently 13 participating units within the Network working with the NICHD, the FDA and the pharmaceutical industry. The PPRU Network has become a valuable resource for studies conducted in children. It has access to approximately 177 000 children who are inpatients and 2 million who are outpatients annually (Paediatric Pharmacology Research Unit Network, 2006).

Regulatory changes in Europe and the UK

Countries in Europe, particularly the UK, are following the positive steps of the USA; a number of regulatory proposals and initiatives have been carried out in an effort to deal with the lack of drug information and dosage forms for children.

In 1997, the European Agency for the Evaluation of Medicinal Products (EMEA, 1997) published a guidance document on the clinical investigation of medicinal products in children. The guidance document encourages and facilitates timely testing of medicines in children by the pharmaceutical industry. The document provided guidance and detailed approaches to the safe, efficient and ethical study of medicinal products in children. Unfortunately it does not carry any legislative authority and concerns have been raised that the release of the guideline may not have resulted in much change.

In December 2000, the European Union Council invited the European Commission to find solutions for the inadequacy of children's medicine research. Hence in 2004, the European Commission adopted a proposal for a Regulation of the Council and of the European Parliament on medicinal products for paediatric use (Commission of the European Communities, 2004). The final version of the text of the Regulation has been agreed by the Council and the European Parliament in 2006. The Regulation aims to establish a legislative framework that will:

1.   Increase the availability of medicines specifically adapted and licensed for use in children.
2.   Increase the information available to the patient/carer and prescriber about the use of medicines in children, including clinical trial data.
3.   Lead to an increase in high-quality research into medicines for children.

The Regulation is very similar to the US regulation, as summarised below:

1.   For patented medicines:
      (a)   A requirement at the time of marketing authorisation applications for new medicines for the inclusion of data on the use of the medicine in children, or a waiver from the requirement for medicines unlikely to benefit children, or a deferral of the requirement to ensure that medicines are tested in children only when it is safe to do so and to prevent the requirements delaying the authorisation of medicines for adults.
      (b)   Medicines (excludes orphan medicines, which are classified under a different reward scheme) that comply with the requirement will be awarded a 6-month patent extension on the active moiety.
2.   For off-patent medicines: a new type of marketing authorisation, the Paediatric Use Marketing Authorisation (PUMA), allows 10 years of data protection for new studies on off-patent products.
3.   The establishment of the Paediatric Committee within the EMEA. The Paediatric Committee will have expertise in all aspects of research, development, authorisation and use of medicines in children.
4.   The accessibility to a EU network of investigators and trial centres so as to facilitate the conduct of children's medicines research.
5.   Enhanced safety monitoring for medicines marketed for children.
6.   Free scientific advice for the pharmaceutical industry from the EMEA.
7.   Information tools, such as an inventory of the therapeutic needs of children and a database of paediatric studies.

Research capacity building

Drug Investigation in Children Network

In 1998 a group of paediatricians and clinical pharmacologists with an interest in paediatric patients collaborated to form the European Network for Drug Investigation in Children (ENDIC) (Van den Anker and Choonara, 1999). ENDIC included researchers from countries such as the Netherlands, France, Germany, Italy, Sweden, Finland, the UK and Israel. The main limitation with this initiative, however, was the absence of funding, in contrast to the US PPRU Network.

Task-force in Europe for Drug Development for the Young Network

In 2005, the Task-force in Europe for Drug Development for the Young (TEDDY, 2006) received funding from the EU Commissioner to set up an EU network research project involving 17 research institutions from 11 countries. Its aim is to improve the paediatric use of current drugs and promote the development of new drugs, by incorporating pharmacogenetic applications and implementing guidance/tools to perform paediatric research.

The following are the objectives of TEDDY:

*   To establish a rationale for the safe and efficacious use of medicines in male/female children based on an understanding of developmental biology, pharmacogenetics and pharmacogenomics.
*   To identify unmet needs for the development and use of medicinal products and orphan drugs in male/female children.
*   To develop, validate and harmonise preclinical and clinical methods for assessing the safety and efficacy of current and new drugs in male/female children.
*   To explore, validate and consolidate the existing data sources containing information on medicines used in male/female children before setting up a harmonised, integrated and reliable European database (or system of databases) to provide an information centre service.
*   To increase awareness of, and contribute to the debate on, the ethical issues arising from paediatric drug research and use (including off-label and unlicensed use), and the extended use of biotechnology for diagnostic and therapeutic purposes.
*   To bring together industries and other relevant stakeholders to encourage the development of new drugs, optimise paediatric

formulations and provide labelling recommendations for current drugs.

- To build critical mass capacity by means of training and education activities, the dissemination of information and the development of guidelines.

At the time of writing this chapter (October 2006), the EMEA is in the process of setting up an EU network of investigators and trial centres so as to facilitate the conduct of children's medicines research as proposed by the Better Medicines for Children regulation (Commission of the European Communities, 2004).

UK Medicines for Children Research Network

The UK Clinical Research Network (UKCRN) was developed in the UK to support clinical research and to facilitate the conduct of randomised prospective trials of interventions and other well-designed studies. It currently supports six topic-specific clinical research networks in the fields of cancer, dementias and neurodegenerative disease, diabetes, medicines for children, mental health and stroke (UK Clinical Research Network, 2006).

A consortium led by the University of Liverpool and Royal Liverpool Children's Hospital have established the Coordinating Centre for the Medicines for Children Research Network (MCRN) (UK Medicines for Children Research Network, 2006). The MCRN aims provide a world-class health service infrastructure to support clinical paediatric research and remove barriers to its conduct.

The MCRN will provide some of the dedicated research resources and staff (£20 million over 5 years) needed to support high-quality, randomised trials of medicines for children and other well-designed research studies.

It is anticipated that the funding available from the MCRN to support the local research networks (LRNs) will be in the region of £500 000 per annum. These resources will provide some of the managerial, administrative and service support costs to support high-quality multicentre studies within the MCRN.

Prescribing information initiatives

Lack of information in paediatric prescribing has long been a problem for clinicians and pharmacists. In order to tackle this problem, in 1999, the Royal College of Paediatrics and Child Health (RCPCH) and the Neonatal and Paediatric Pharmacists Group (NPPG) published the first edition of *Medicines for Children* formulary (Neonatal and Paediatric Pharmacists Group, 2006). It contains information on general guidance prescribing in children, and details individual drug information and nutritional information for a selection of formulas and nutritional supplements. *Medicines for Children* has been an important resource for prescribing since it was launched and the second edition was published in 2003.

The successful partnership between the RCPCH and NPPG further extended to the *British National Formulary* (BNF) (jointly published by British Medical Association and Royal Pharmaceutical Society of Great Britain). The *British National Formulary for Children* (BNFC) was launched in the UK in 2005 (*BNF for Children*, 2006). The BNFC covers newborn babies to 18 year olds and gives a range of guidance, from choosing the best available drug to specific doses and formulations. The UK Department of Health invested £1.8 million in the BNFC project and 175 000 copies of the BNFC are provided free of charge for doctors and other prescribers of paediatric medicines in the NHS. As with the BNF, it is expected that the BNFC will be used world-wide and will certainly be the most widely used paediatric prescribing reference.

References

BNF for Children (2006). http://bnfc.org/bnfc/ (accessed January 2006).

Commission of the European Communities (2004). Proposal for a regulation of the European Parliament and of the Council on medicinal products for paediatric use and amending regulation (EEC) No 1768/92, Directive 2001/83/EC and Regulation (EC) No 726/2004. Brussels.

Department of Health and Human Services (2001). The pediatric exclusivity provision – January 2001 status report to congress. Food and Drug Administration, 2001. http://www.fda.gov/cder/pediatric/reportcong01.pdf (accessed January 2006).

European Agency for the Evaluation of Medicinal Products (EMEA) (1997). *Note for Guidance on Clinical Investigation of Medicinal Products in Children.* London: EMEA.

Food and Drug Administration (1994). Specific requirements on content and format of labeling for human prescription drugs; revision of 'pediatric use' subsection in the labeling; final rule, 21 CFR Part 201 (December 13, 1994). http://www.fda.gov/cder/pediatric/pediatric_rule1994.htm (accessed January 2006).

Food and Drug Administration (1997). Food and Drug Administration Modernization Act of 1997, Public Law. No. 105–115 (November 21, 1997). http://www.fda.gov/cder/guidance/105-115.htm#SEC.%20111 (accessed January 2006).

Food and Drug Administration (1998). 21 CFR Parts 201, 312, 314, and 601 [Docket No. 97N-0165] RIN 0910-AB20 Regulations Requiring Manufacturers to Assess the Safety and Effectiveness of New Drugs and Biological Products in Pediatric Patients (December 2, 1998). http://www.fda.gov/cder/guidance/pedrule.htm (accessed January 2006).

Food and Drug Administration (2002). Best Pharmaceuticals for Children Act. Public Law 107–109 (January 4, 2002). http://www.fda.gov/opacom/laws/pharmkids/contents.html (accessed January 2006).

Food and Drug Administration (2003). The Pediatric Research Equity Act. Public Law 108–155 (December 3, 2003). http://www.fda.gov/cder/pediatric/S-650-PREA.pdf (accessed January 2006).

Neonatal and Paediatric Pharmacists Group (2006). *Medicines For Children*, 2nd edn. http://www.nppg.org.uk/ (accessed January 2006).

Pediatric Pharmacology Research Unit Network (2006). http://www.ppru.org/ (accessed January 2006).

Task-force in Europe for Drug Development for the Young (TEDDY) (2006). http://www.teddyoung.org/ (accessed January 2006).

UK Clinical Research Network (2006). http://www.ukcrn.org.uk/ (accessed January 2006).

UK Medicines for Children Research Network (2006). http://www.liv.ac.uk/mcrn/index2.htm (accessed January 2006).

van den Anker J, Choonara I (1999). ENDIC European Network for Drug Investigation in Children. *Paediatr Perinat Drug Ther* 3: 15–16.

Wong I, Sweis D, Cope J, *et al.* (2003). Paediatric medicines research in the UK: How to move forward? *Drug Safety* 26: 529–537.

6

Clinical trials in children

Vincent Yeung

Ethics and recruitment issues

Evidence-based medicine and healthcare are the pillar of optimal medical care. However, there are deficits in our understanding of the quality and efficacy of paediatric therapies, many of which are based on anecdotal data and evidence. Over 50% of medicines used in children are not licensed for use either for the disease states or for the age group. The extrapolation of adult data on medicinal products for the child population is inappropriate, which makes age- and development-related research particularly important. The need to develop medicines in children, whether it is a novel agent or an existing agent in need of pharmacokinetic study, necessitates testing on children. The promise of making drugs safer for children increases the potential for harm to children who serve as research participants. Sometimes it is difficult, if not impossible, to quantify the risk. Without knowing the nature of future risks, to what extent can permission be given to child participation in clinical research? Researchers need to consider the ethical issues of conducting clinical trials in children, not only on a theoretical level, but also on a practical level in the form of ethical approval and statutory requirements.

The most commonly performed clinical trials evaluate new medical therapies on patients in strictly scientifically controlled settings. The purpose of such trials is to determine whether one or more treatment options are safe, effective and better than current standard care. Controlled trials require a higher standard of consent than treating patients unsystematically. Ethically, it is more justifiable to conduct controlled trials than treatments based on anecdotal evidence, as the controlled trial is more likely to clarify the efficacy and safety of a new treatment and its adverse effects.

Patients enrolled in clinical trials are more likely to be benefited by the 'inclusion effect' (Lantos, 1999). Babies who received placebo in a placebo-controlled trial of antithrombin therapy in neonatal respiratory distress syndrome, for example, had a significantly shorter mean duration of ventilation than non-randomised babies. This could be explained by the more vigorous observations and monitoring as prescribed by the protocol.

Beauchamp and Childress (2001) advocate four principles – autonomy, beneficence, non-maleficence and justice – to form the basis of bioethics discussion. However, in paediatric research, the model of 'best interests of the child' sets a paradigm of a combination of parental consent and assents by the child as advocated in the Belmont Report (1978) in the USA.

Clinical research in the UK is governed by statutory requirements in the form of the EU Directive (2001/20/EC) on Good Clinical Practice (GCP), ethical principles (Declaration of Helsinki), the Research Governance Framework for Health and Social Care (Department of Health, 2005) and the duty of care in the National Health Service (NHS), the high professional and ethical standards that most care professionals and researchers uphold.

Declaration of Helsinki

In 1964, the World Medical Association established a statement of ethical principles to provide guidance to physicians and other participants in biomedical research involving humans. It was developed to correct the perceived deficiencies in the Nuremberg Code, especially on physician-led research with patients. The Declaration governs international research ethics and defines rules for 'research combined with clinical care' and 'non-therapeutic research'. The Declaration of Helsinki was revised in 1975, 1983, 1989 and 1996 and is the basis for GCP used today. A summarised version of the Declaration of Helsinki is shown in Table 6.1.

The Declaration of Helsinki has considerable influence in the field of ethics in biomedical research and forms the basis of GCP and subsequent legislation in European Economic Area (EEA) countries. The latest EU GCP Directive (2005/28/EC) has specified the use of the 1996 version of the Declaration.

History of good clinical practice

Good clinical practice (GCP) is a formal approach to the procedures applied to various stages of clinical trials. A summary of the history of

Table 6.1 Summary of the Declaration of Helsinki 1996

I. **Basic principles**
 1. Biomedical research must conform to generally accepted scientific principles and should be based on adequately performed laboratory and animal experimentation and on a thorough knowledge of the scientific literature.
 2. Protocols should be clear and reviewed independently and must conform to the laws and regulations of the country in which the research experiment is performed.
 3. Medical research should be conducted by scientifically qualified persons and supervised by a clinical qualified person.
 4. Biomedical research cannot legitimately be carried out unless the importance of the objective is in proportion to the inherent risk to the subject.
 5. Concern for the interests of the subject must always prevail over the interests of science and society.
 6. The right of the research subject and his or her integrity must always be respected.
 7. Predictable risk and investigation should cease if the hazards are found to outweigh the potential benefits.
 8. Accuracy of the results and reports should only be accepted when research is conducted in accordance with the principles laid down in this Declaration.
 9. Subjects must be adequately informed of the aim, methods, benefits and potential risks of the study and the discomfort it may entail. Subjects should be informed of their right to refuse to participate and the right to withdraw at any time.
 10. Patients should not give consent under duress or be influenced by the dependent relationship with physicians.
 11. Informed consent should be obtained from legal guardians for minors and mentally incapable adults; if possible, minors should give assent.
 12. The research protocol should always contain a statement of the ethical considerations and compliance with the Declaration.

II. **Medical research combined with professional care (clinical research)**
 1. A physician must be free to use a new diagnostic and therapeutic measure, if it offers hope of saving life, reestablishing health or alleviating suffering of the patient.
 2. The potential benefits, hazards and discomfort of a new method should be weighed against the advantages of the best current diagnostic and therapeutic methods.
 3. Every patient, including the control group, should receive the best proven diagnostic and therapeutic method. This does not exclude the use of inert placebo in studies where no proven diagnostic or therapeutic method exists.
 4. The refusal of the patient to participate in a study must never interfere with the physician–patient relationship.
 5. If the informed consent is not taken, the specific reasons should be stated in the protocol and be approved by an independent committee.
 6. The physician can combine medical research with professional care. Medical research is justified by its potential diagnostic or therapeutic value for the patient.

continued

Table 6.1 Continued

III. Non-therapeutic biomedical research involving human subjects (non-clinical biomedical research)

1. In the purely scientific application, it is the duty of the physician to remain the protector of the life and health of that person on whom biomedical research is being carried out.
2. The subjects should be volunteers – either healthy persons or patients for whom the experimental design is not related to the patient's illness.
3. The investigator or the investigating team should discontinue the research if in his or her or their judgement it may, if continued, be harmful to the individual.
4. In research on humans, the interest of science and society should never take precedence over considerations related to the well-being of the subject.

---

the development of GCP legislation and guidelines is shown in Table 6.2. GCP is an international standard governing the design, conduct, recording and reporting of clinical trials. It has gestated through years of accidents in the history of medicines and violation of human rights in the name of biomedical research. In 1947 through the Nuremberg Code, the principle of informed consent was established. The Code was the result of the unethical clinical experiments conducted with war prisoners during World War II. The thalidomide incidents in the late 1950s and early 1960s led to the formation of the Committee of the Safety of Medicines in 1964 in the UK and the requirement for the licensing of medicinal products was issued by the EU (65/65/EC) for all the member states. In response, the UK Government issued the Medicinal Act in 1968 and the Good Manufacturing Practice (GMP) Inspectorate was set up.

In 1975 an EU Directive (75/318/EEC) required each member state to ensure the submission of safety and efficacy for marketing authorisation. Good laboratory practice (GLP) became the principle of non-clinical testing on pharmaceutical products and the requirement of a GCP standard in conducting clinical trials. It stated that 'all phases of clinical investigation, including bioavailability and bioequivalence studies shall be designed, implemented and reported in accordance of GCP' (75/318/EEC, B.1.1).

In July 1991, the European Commission published the Enforcement of the EEC Note for Guidance: 'Good Clinical Practice for Trials on Medicinal Products in the European Community'. This enforcement was setting into operation GCP guidelines that were, however, not yet legally binding at that time. Directive 91/507/EEC was published to modify the annex to Council Directive 75/318/EEC. By this enforcement

Table 6.2 History of good clinical practice (GCP) and related legislation and directives

Year	Event	Comment
1947	Nuremberg Code	Principle of informed consent
1964 (revised 1975, 1983, 1989, 1996)	Declaration of Helsinki	
1965	65/65/EC	Licensing of medicinal product
1968	Medicinal Act	
1975	75/318/EEC	Safety and efficacy requirement for marketing authorisation. GLP became the principle of non-clinical testing
1991	91/507/EEC	GCP in EEC
1997	CPMP/ICH/135/95	ICH GCP published by Committee for Proprietary Medicinal Products
2001	2001/20 EC	EU Clinical Trial Directive
2001	2001/83/EC (part 4, B1)	Community code on medicinal product, requirement of GCP in conducting clinical trials
2003	2003/63/EC	Amendment on 2001/83/EC. Part 1, 5.2.c defines holding period of essential clinical trials document
2003	2003/94/EC	GMP requirements for IMP
2003	EUDRACT	EUDRACT database guidance note
2003	Annex 13	Manufacture of IMPs
2004	2004/27/EC (13)	GCP requirement for clinical trials outside the EEA
2004	SI 2004/1031	The Medicines for Human Use (Clinical Trials) Regulation's 2004
2005	2005/28/EC	Guidelines for GCP
2006	SI 2006/1928	The Medicines for Human Use (Clinical Trials) Amendment Regulation's 2006

EEA, European Economic Area; GLP, good laboratory practice; GMP, good manufacturing practice; ICH, International Conference on Harmonisation; IMP, investigational medicinal product; SI, statutory instruments.

the European member states were obliged to bring into force the laws, regulations and administrative provisions necessary to comply with the Directive that requests – besides others – all clinical trials to be designed, implemented and recorded in accordance with GCP.

In 1996 the International Conference on Harmonisation (ICH) issued a guideline for GCP (E6) (ICH, 1996). This was instigated by the desire to promote international consensus on mutual recognition of clinical trials and marketing authorisation procedure. This was adopted by the Committee for Proprietary Medicinal Products (CPMP, now CHMP) and formally accepted as the standard in the EU in 1997, replacing the previous EU GCP guideline.

Directive 2001/20/EC of the European Parliament and of the Council of 4 April 2001, on the approximation of the laws, regulations and administrative provisions of the member states, relates to the implementation of GCP in the conduct of clinical trials on medicinal products for human use. The community code relating to medicinal products for human use (2001/83/EC) was amended in 2003 (2003/63/EC), stipulating that clinical trials data used for marketing authorisation applications in the EU are required to be conducted in accordance with GCP.

The year 2003 saw the launch of the European Clinical Trials (EudraCT) Database (https://eudract.emea.eu.int/eudract/index.do). The database is interfaced with the Eudravigilance Clinical Trial Module (EVCTM), and is used to facilitate communication on clinical trials between authorities in the oversight of clinical trials and investigational medicinal product development, and to provide for enhanced protection of clinical trial participants receiving investigational medicinal products.

In the UK SI 2004 1031 was implemented, incorporating into British law the requirement of the EU Directive 2001/20/EC. Finally the EU-issued Directive 2005/28/EC, which lays down principles and detailed guidelines for GCP in investigational medicinal products for human use and the requirements for authorisation of the manufacturing of investigational medicinal products, required member states to implement it into law by 29 January 2006. In the UK, the GCP Directive was implemented in August 2006.

Implication of the legislation

The development of GCP from an international guideline to a statutory requirement has caused upheaval in academic research. Before the legislation, academic research involving already marketed products and not intended to generate results for marketing authorisation purpose was exempt from these rules. Now, however, all research involving humans and investigational medicinal products is covered by the legislation, and publicly funded clinical trials must fulfil the same requirements as their commercial counterparts. It is the responsibility of the sponsor to ensure that clinical trials are designed, conducted, recorded and reported in accordance with GCP standards.

To comply with the new legislation the sponsor needs to develop a set of standard operation procedures (SOPs) to cover all areas of trial activities. A quality system should be in place to ensure record-keeping and verification of data entry or extraction of data from the case report form (CRF), capture adverse events (AEs), serious adverse events (SAEs) and unexpected serious adverse reactions (SUSARs) and report in an expedited manner data transfer from source data to database and archiving of the source data for audit purpose. GCP and trial specific training should be carried out and recorded in a timely manner.

Ethics committee

An ethics committee is an independent body constituted of medical/scientific professionals and non-scientific members, whose responsibility is to ensure the protection of the rights, safety and well-being of humans involved in a trial. It provides public assurance of that protection by, among other things, reviewing and approving/providing favourable opinion on the trial protocol, the suitability of the investigator(s), facilities, and the methods and material to be used in obtaining and documenting informed consent of the trial participants.

In the UK, the United Kingdom Ethics Committees Authority (UKECA) is responsible for establishing, recognising and monitoring ethics committees. The Authority may establish ethics committees to act for the entire UK or for each area of the UK and the description or class of clinical trial in relation to which it may act. The categories are listed in Table 6.3.

Clinical trials of medicinal products for gene therapy are subject to separate arrangements for ethical review. Applications relating to such trials should be submitted to the Gene Therapy Advisory

Table 6.3 Types of ethics committee in the UK

Types of ethic committees	Expertise
1	Phase I clinical trials of medicinal products in healthy volunteers throughout the UK
2	Investigational medicinal products (other than phase I trials in healthy volunteers) to take place only at sites within an area defined by the geographical remit of their own appointing authority
3	As in type 2 but at any site in the UK

Committee (GTAC), which is recognised as a specialist committee by UKECA under the Clinical Trials Regulations.

The 'main research ethics committee (REC)' is the REC that undertakes the ethical review of an application. All subsequent amendments should be reviewed by the main REC. An application for ethical review of a research study should be made by the chief investigator for that study. Applications may not be submitted by the sponsor(s) on behalf of the chief investigator. Only one application for ethical review should be submitted in relation to any research protocol to be conducted within the UK. In the case of international studies, an application must be made to an ethics committee in the UK, whether or not the study has a favourable ethical opinion from a committee outside the UK and whether or not it has started outside the UK. Trials of medicinal products that are 'non-interventional' are not classified as clinical trials of an investigational medicinal product (CTIMPs) and do not require review by a recognised REC. If in doubt about the classification of a trial, it is the responsibility of the chief investigator or sponsor to seek authoritative advice from the Medicines and Healthcare products Regulatory Agency (MHRA).

Under the clinical trials regulations, an REC is required to give an ethical opinion on an application relating to a CTIMP within 60 calendar days of the receipt of a valid application. Where the REC considers that further information is required in order to give an opinion, the REC may make one request in writing for further information from the applicant. The period of 60 days will be suspended pending receipt of this information.

Where a study involves certain types of research procedure, the suitability of each site or sites at which the research is to be conducted requires 'site-specific assessment' (SSA). The SSA is not a separate ethical review, but forms part of the single ethical review of the research. Where there is no objection on site-specific grounds, a site may be approved as part of the favourable ethical opinion given by the main REC. When submitting an application, the chief investigator should declare if in his or her opinion the research does not require SSA at any research site. Where such a declaration is made, this should be considered by the main REC at the meeting at which the application is ethically reviewed.

Non-therapeutic research

The Royal College of Paediatrics and Child Health guidelines (2000) indicate that a research procedure that is not intended directly to benefit the child is not necessarily either unethical or illegal. Research work can offer valuable training that may improve the quality of doctors' clinical practice. However, research that could equally well be done on adults should never be done on children. Non-therapeutic research on children should not carry greater than minimal risk of harm. Second, the risks posed by non-therapeutic procedures should be proportional to the knowledge that may reasonably be expected to be gained.

Some research based on observation, collating information from notes and tests already performed for therapeutic purposes, may be permissible without consent because it does not involve direct contact with the child. Researchers must be careful in this matter and consult the Central Office for Research Ethics Committees (COREC) to ascertain this requirement. Non-therapeutic research can be validly consented only when the research can be reasonably said not to go against the child's interests. Even though it is not legally required, research should seek assent from school-age children and should always ensure that the child does not object.

Informed consent

The informed consent process is the foundation of any ethical research. Researchers should have a clear understanding of the process on a theoretical and practical level to conduct ethics studies, to improve parents'/patients' understanding and expectation, and to improve recruitment rates.

Article 3 of 2005/28/EC stipulates that clinical trials shall be conducted in accordance with the Declaration of Helsinki on ethical principles for medical research involving humans adopted by the General Assembly at the World Medical Association in 1996. Principle 9 states that:

> In any research on human beings, each potential subject must be adequately informed of the aims, methods, anticipated benefits and potential hazards of the study and the discomfort it may entail. He or she should be informed that he or she is at liberty to abstain from participation in the study and that he or she is free to withdraw his or her consent to participation at any time.

In other words, the participant should have adequate knowledge and understanding to participate in research, whether it is diagnostic, therapeutic or a preventive intervention. The understanding includes why the research is being done, what will be done during the trial and for how long, what risks are involved, what, if any, benefit can be expected from the trial and, more importantly, what other interventions are available.

The participant also has the right to leave the trial at any time without giving the reason and without giving up their legal rights. Informed consent should be documented by means of a signed, dated, informed consent form, preferably witnessed by a third party who is not part of the clinical trial team.

The purpose of informed consent is to ensure that individuals have control over whether or not to enrol in clinical research and to ensure that they participate only when the research is consistent with their values, interests and preferences. The decision of an individual should be rational, free, voluntary and uncoerced. Children who are unable to make their own decisions also have interests and values. Their preferences and values may be unknown or unknowable. In such cases, research proxy is used to determine whether to enrol them in clinical research.

In the case of minors, Principle 11 of the Declaration of Helsinki stipulates that 'permission from the responsible relative replaces that of the subject in accordance with national legislation'. SI 2004 1031 Schedule 1 Part 4.1 stipulates that a person with parental responsibility can give informed consent on behalf of a minor. Mothers always have parental responsibility. Unmarried fathers do not automatically have parental responsibility for their children. An unmarried father can acquire parental responsibility by: applying for and getting a residence order or parental responsibility order; making a parental responsibility agreement (in a set procedure) with the mother; being appointed the child's guardian (once the appointment takes effect); or subsequently marrying the mother of the child. A step-parent may acquire parental responsibility by obtaining a Residence Order or adopting the child. The different regulations, directives and standards on informed consent for minors are compared in Table 6.4.

The informed consent process

Some have argued that the informed consent process for complex clinical trials can give rise to misunderstanding and feelings of powerlessness, especially for those who are poorly educated and emotionally stressed (Mason, 1997). There is also a tendency for some doctors to avoid the consent issue because they want to 'protect' the patient. In one recent report about the Continuous Negative Extrathoracic Pressure (CNEP) trial, doctors were said to have 'sold' a trial to patients as a 'kinder, gentler treatment' without telling them that they were participating in a clinical trial (Smith, 2000).

Table 6.4 Informed consent requirements of various guidelines, directives and regulations for minors participating in clinical research

Requirements	SI 2004 1031[a]	Directive 2001/20/EC[b]	ICH GCP E6 1997[c]	Declaration of Helsinki 1996[d]
A legal representative for the minor must have an interview with the investigator and has been given the opportunity to understand the objectives, risks and inconveniences of the trial and the conditions under which it is to be conducted	Schedule 1 Part 4.1		4.8.5	9
The legal representative has been informed of the right to withdraw the minor from the trial at any time	Schedule 1 Part 4.3	Article 4.a	4.8.10	9
The legal representative has given his or her informed consent	Schedule 1 Part 4.4	Article 4.a	4.8.5	11
The minor has received information according to his or her capacity for understanding from staff with experience with minors, the trial's risk and its benefits	Schedule 1 Part 4.6	Article 4.b	4.8.12	
A minor who is capable of forming an opinion must give assent to the trial and can withdraw at any time	Schedule 1 Part 4.7	Article 4.c	4.8.12	11
The clinical trial relates directly to a clinical condition from which the minor suffers or is of such a nature that it can be carried out only on minors	Schedule 1 Part 4.9	Article 4.e		
Some direct benefit is to be obtained	Schedule 1 Part 4.10			
The corresponding scientific guidelines of the European Medicines Agency are followed	Schedule 1 Part 4.12	Article 4.f		
The clinical trial has been designed to minimise pain, discomfort, fear and any other foreseeable risk in relation to the disease and the minor's stage of development	Schedule 1 Part 4.14	Article 4.g		
The Ethics Committee, with paediatric expertise or after taking advice in clinical, ethical and psychological problems in the field of paediatrics, has endorsed the protocol		Article 4.h		
The interests of the patient always prevail over those of science and society	Schedule 1 Part 4.16	Article 4.i	2.3	5

[a]SI 2004 1031 The Medicines for Human Use (Clinical Trials) Regulation 2004.
[b]EC/2001/20 Official Journal L121, 1/5/2001 pp. 34–44.
[c]ICH E6 1997 CPMP/ICH/135/95.
[d]Declaration of Helsinki 48th WMA General Assembly, Somerset West, Republic of South Africa, October 1996.

Parents do not always remember that they have given consent to a study. A small proportion of parents (2.5%) in the Euricon study could not remember being asked to give consent (Mason and Allmark, 2000), and, in another study, the figure was as high as 12% (Stenson *et al.*, 2004). Some parents do not think that there is adequate discussion of alternatives to proposed novel treatments and the scope of the research protocol. This is a common issue with paediatric oncology trials where most treatments are protocol driven (Kupst *et al.*, 2003).

One study found that a high proportion (25%) of parents felt obliged to participate (van Stuijvenberg *et al.*, 1998). This may be due to a feeling of being dependent on the investigator or the hospital. Parents who feel obliged to consent are classed as having failed the informed consent procedure, because they have not truly given informed consent.

Parents may experience guilt for not making the right decision, especially when a baby dies. The process may coerce people into participating or they may be influenced by the desire for a particular treatment that is unavailable in normal circumstance. In neonatal research, the mother may be exhausted or with impaired cognitive function due to a sedative or analgesia. Their worry is exasperated by the admission of uncertainty that leads to the research in the first place. The post-trial interview of parents whose children had undergone the UK extracorporeal membrane oxygenation (ECMO) trial expresses their sense of fear and haste when they were approached by the researchers. They were also angry and distressed when their babies were randomised to conventional treatment (Snowdon *et al.*, 1997).

Researchers should understand the dynamic of parental thought processes. Ample time and sufficient but not overwhelming information should be given to parents to decide whether to allow their children to take part in the study. They should see the giving of informed consent as a process, not as an event; regular updates and reinforcement increase parental understanding and facilitate continuous participation.

Assent and age

Parental consent will probably be invalid if it is given against the child's interests.

It is completely inappropriate to insist on the taking of blood for non-therapeutic reasons if a child indicates either significant unwillingness before the start or significant stress during the procedure.

At what patient age should the researcher ask for assent? The ICH does not yield any answers; the phrase 'if capable' does not give us any guidance. In reality, there is no such benchmark for minimal chronological age, but it depends on the perceived maturity and the degree of understanding (Rossi *et al.*, 2003). Some suggest that researchers should give more weight to parental consent in therapeutic research but even more to a child's dissent for non-therapeutic research (Barfield and Church, 2005). The law in the UK concerning research on children has never been clearly established. The law requires a child who has 'sufficient understanding and intelligence to understand what is proposed' to give consent (*Gillick v West Norfolk* 1985).

Researchers should engage young children by providing them with information appropriate to their level of understanding. Young children with long-term illnesses have a better understanding of their conditions and the concept of research than their older counterparts who have little exposure to a hospital environment or medical research. Despite parental consent, researchers should respect the will of the children when they decline to take part in a study.

Consent process in emergency

In the case of an emergency, and when the person with parental responsibility is not contactable prior to the inclusion of the participant in the trial, a legal representative for the minor can give informed consent. In the UK, that will be someone other than the person involved in the conduct of the trial, who by virtue of his or her relationship with that minor is suitable to act as a legal representative for the purposes of the trial and is available and willing to act for those purposes. When no such person is available, a doctor who is primarily responsible for the medical treatment provided to the child, and is not connected to the clinical trial, can act as a professional representative. It is possible, however, that it would still be unlawful if the research were not expected to benefit the child in question.

Fast decision-making is crucial in an emergency; it has been argued that reasonable understanding and voluntariness are likely to be severely compromised (Hewlett, 1996; Manning, 2000). In many neonatal scenarios such as resuscitation, surfactant treatment, modes of respiratory support, treatment of seizures, little time is available for parents to decide participation in clinical trials.

There are alternative approaches that avoid taking consent (Modi, 1994). For example, researchers can discuss the study with parents antenatally. Then when the child is born and is eligible for the study, the parents are asked whether they would like to opt out of the research. If there is no objection, their babies will be automatically enrolled in the study. Support for such an approach comes from studies that demonstrate that a significant minority of parents would prefer to have their doctor advise them on whether to include their baby in neonatal research than have to decide themselves (Zupancic *et al.*, 1997). The downside is that it may override the autonomy of the parents, but this can be mitigated by continuous communication and information sharing and consents for non-therapeutics and non-urgent research should still be sought (Manning, 2000).

Presumed consent is another option where antenatal consent is sought from parents (Morley, 1997). It is particular useful in situations where obtaining conventional consent is impractical. It should be supplemented by informing parents as soon as possible and obtaining 'continuous consent' while the baby is still in the trial. The criticism of such an approach is that parents may pay little heed to trial information given antenatally, assuming that their baby is unlikely to be affected.

It has been argued that the opting-out processes would protect vulnerable and deprived families who are less capable of understanding the rationale of the research and consent processes and are likely to give consent and participate in research. The opt-out process will allow these families to participate and reduce selection bias, thus producing more generalisable conclusions and being more equitable (Rogers *et al.*, 1998; Manning, 2000). However, the legality of such approaches in drug trials needs to be explored in view of the latest regulations. Moreover, it has been demonstrated that 83% of parents who consented did not want to forego the consent process, and only 8% of the respondents were unhappy about giving consent (Stenson *et al.*, 2004). In one post-trial interview, 98% of parents with babies in a neonatal intensive care unit wanted to decide and did not want doctors or nurses to decide (Morley, 2004).

Parental understanding of randomisation

The prerequisite for an ethical randomised control trial is that it provides no certain benefit to the individual patients and in fact could harm the child as the result of potential side effects. Research is justified when there is no convincing ground that any patient would be advantaged or disadvantaged if allocated to one treatment arm over the others (Freedman, 1987a). It has been shown that research participants often fail to understand that their treatment has been selected at random

(Edwards *et al.*, 1998). For example, 74% of the patients attending an oncology clinic thought that their doctor would ensure that they received the best treatment offered in randomised clinical trial (Ellis *et al.*, 1999). Again, in the ECMO study, some parents believed that randomisation meant rationing access or a solution to difficult clinical decision-making (Snowdon *et al.*, 1997). In contrast, 88% of parents were aware that their children might receive a placebo in a double-blind study of ibuprofen in the prevention of recurrent febrile seizures (van Stuijvenberg *et al.*, 1998). These diverse observations may be attributed to differences in the complexity and nature of the studies, educational background and the state of mind of the parents.

For the very reason that public understanding is low, some researchers suggest using 'by chance' or 'by the flip of a coin' instead (Waggoner and Mayo, 1995). COREC guidelines suggest that the phrase 'The groups are selected by a computer which has no information about the individual' should be used (COREC, 2006). A more solid approach to ascertain participants' understanding is to allow them to demonstrate explicit understanding by giving a verbal definition of randomisation.

Methods to improve the informed consent process

The deficiency in patients' understanding of the consent process is apparent; many have called for investigators and institutions to take action to improve research participants' understanding (Lavori *et al.*, 1999; Siminoff, 2003). A systematic review has shown that five main categories of interventions have been used (Flory and Emanuel, 2004). These include multimedia, enhanced consent forms, extended discussion and test/feedback. In 12 trials, multimedia interventions, including video or computer presentation, failed to improve research participants' understanding. Multimedia may be a way to standardise disclosure but it does not add much to the standard disclosure procedure.

Improved presentation in consent forms such as changing the format, font size and adding graphics had little effect, but a shortened form and the removal of irrelevant information did have a significant improvement. When designing a patient information leaflet it should be remembered that quantitative information is often difficult for the general public to understand (Schwartz *et al.*, 1997). Probabilistic language troubles many individuals, and parents and clinicians prefer to use relative rather than absolute terms in assessing risks and benefits (Forrow *et al.*, 1992). Researchers should use simple words, avoiding medical jargon, and sentences should be short (Tarnowski *et al.*, 1990).

Extended discussion between staff and research participants and the test/feedback approach had a significant impact on understanding. But the use of small sample sizes and methodological flaws may not provide enough evidence to support their validity. The rationale of using these approaches is that active engagement and responsiveness to the individual participants of research may improve understanding. The informed consent process is not merely reading and signing a form, but it is a continuous dialogue and takes place over time.

Enrolling patients in multiple trials

Many ethics committee consider it inappropriate for patients to be asked to consent to join more than one study. It is not uncommon for patients with childhood leukaemia to be approached for numerous studies looking at different initial regimens, genetic studies for the family or the disease cells, or psychosocial studies looking at how families cope with long-term illness. The argument for involving certain patients in several studies is that some diseases, such as cystinosis or urea cycle defects, are very rare and it is impossible to recruit all the sufferers in the world. To restrict such patients will result in fewer interventions being evaluated (Brocklehurst, 1994) and treating patients without assessing the risks and benefits of a certain treatment is equally unethical. The counter-argument is that the extra blood samples and visits required by the study procedures create an unnecessary burden on families who are barely able to cope with their diseases. This is more so when the outcome of the studies may not be beneficial to the participants.

In a survey of parents with preterm infants in the neonatal intensive care unit (NICU) who had been asked to join two or more studies, 58% were willing for their baby to be in three or more studies (Morley *et al.*, 2005). Parents are willing to help other children with similar conditions even though they know that their own children may not benefit from the study. Researchers should exercise their judgement to decide the appropriateness of using the same patient population for different studies. They need to ask: Is this patient population over-researched? Can we make use of a different patient group?

Enrolling children in phase I studies

Phase I studies are usually avoided in paediatrics because the risk to a child is more than minimal. The chance of having a significant clinical response is minimal and it is questionable whether parents are ethically suitable to give permission for their child to be enrolled in such a study. It has been argued that in a palliative care situation, where all possible treatment has failed, it is ethically justifiable to enrol a child into a phase I study if the chance of benefit from the new agent is comparable to that of palliative care or continuation of failed therapy (Barfield and Church, 2005). One would need to justify the extra suffering that may have been incurred with the new therapy, but a well-designed trial can mitigate this (Kodish, 2003).

Factors affecting informed consent

Parents have different reasons for allowing their children to participate in clinical research. A researcher should understand these factors and take them into account in trial design and parent/patient education. The aim is to improve the recruitment rate, on the one hand, and parents'/patients' satisfaction, on the other. Less well-informed parents may misconstrue that their child will get better treatment or will get a novel treatment in a randomised trial and will be disappointed when the result or randomisation does not correspond to their perception. Fundamentally, such a misunderstanding threatens their ability to make an informed choice.

Most studies on parental perception have been carried out within 72 hours of research participation decisions (Zupancic *et al.*, 1997; Hoehn *et al.*, 2005); others are retrospective or prospective questionnaire studies (van Stuijvenberg *et al.*, 1998). Factors that influence parental decisions are societal benefit, personal benefit, risk perception and perceived lack of harm. The logistic factors that influence parental perception of risks are the amount of information given, the trust in the institution and the time required for the decision-making. Parents who perceived benefit, either personal or societal, were more likely to participate than if they perceived risk (Tait *et al.*, 2004; Hoehn *et al.*, 2005). Societal benefit is the most frequently cited reason for participation in clinical research. Parents with a critically ill child have an altruistic view to help future children in similar conditions (Langley *et al.*, 1998; van Stuijvenberg *et al.*, 1998; Schmidt *et al.*, 1999; Mason and Allmark, 2000; Hoehn *et al.*, 2005).

Personal benefit was another common reason. A retrospective survey and prospective interview of parents with children in NICUs has shown that 34–43% of parents had chosen to participate because they believed that their child would get better care in the study (Burgess *et al.*,

2003). Potential benefit may be in the form of increased understanding about their child's disease (Rothmier *et al.*, 2003).

The major factor that influences parental decisions is the perceived risk of the research. It is important to distinguish the risks perceived when considering participation from the risk appreciated while participating in the study. In one study, 74% of parents when asked about hypothetical enrolment of their newborn into a clinical trial refused to participate because of the perceived risk of side effects and the unproved efficacy of the trial medication (Autret *et al.*, 1993). Even the perception of minor risk such as painful procedures may sway parents' choice on participation (Langley *et al.*, 1998).

Those who chose to participate in a research study perceived that there was no risk of harm associated with participation. Parental age affects perceptions of risk: parents who were older (over 30 years) assessed the risks as significantly lower than their younger counterparts (Tait *et al.*, 2004). Furthermore, those who had experience of participation in clinical research had a more positive outlook than those did not have research experience. Sociological factors may have some influence on parental participation in clinical studies. One study has indicated that parents with a higher socioeconomic status and more social support were less motivated to contribute to medical research (Harth and Thong, 1990).

Individuals have different needs of cognition. Parents who perceived that they had been given too much or too little information assessed the risks and benefits more negatively than those who believed they had received just the right amount of information (Tait *et al.*, 2004).

Parents who perceived that they have insufficient time or privacy to make a decision tend to assess the risk and benefit in a more negative light (Hoehn *et al.*, 2005). This is partly a result of stress; parents who were anxious were more likely to decline their child's participation (Tait *et al.*, 2003). This would explain why parents are more likely to give consent in an inpatient setting than in an outpatient preoperative setting (Tait *et al.*, 1998), where there was little time and lack of privacy to ponder the issue. Every effort should be made to provide information in an unhurried manner to alleviate anxiety.

Trust is another important factor affecting the perception of risk by parents. Those who had more trust in the medical system tended to have a more positive outlook on research studies. It is not surprising to discover that individuals from ethic minorities have less trust in research and the medical establishment and are less likely to take part in clinical research (Corbie-Smith *et al.*, 1999; Shavers and Burmeister, 2002).

Application of ethics

For most researchers, the ethics approval process is a daunting path. The successful ethics application starts with a well-written protocol and document control. ICH E6 Section 6 recommends a list of topics that are fundamental for most research (ICH, 1996). A well-written protocol following a template such as background, trial objective, trial design, end-point, statistics and ethics will make the completion of an ethics application form effortless.

All versions of protocols should be version controlled, tracked and retained. The final version should be peer reviewed, approved and signed by the chief investigator. All related documentation, such as patient information sheet (PIS) and informed consent form (ICF), should be version controlled and clearly defined in the ethics application. The ICF should refer to the correct version of the PIS. The ICF should be written in easily understandable language with minimal use of technical terms or languages. Different versions of ICFs should be prepared for parents and for participants with different levels of understanding; usually these are grouped into teenage, older and young children. All other related materials such as letters to GPs, advertising material or questionnaires should also be version controlled or at least have a reference date.

The next step is to identify the sponsor as defined in the Research Governance Framework (Department of Health, 2005) and SI 2004 1031. The identity of the sponsor is required for both the ethics application and EudraCT database. All drug trials should register with the EudraCT database. Where the trial has co-sponsors, these should be identified. The MHRA algorithm (MHRA, 2006) will enable researchers to decide whether the trial is under UK regulation.

The first stage in the EudraCT registration process is to obtain an authenticated security code; this is followed by the EudraCT number and then clinical trial application. The EudraCT database enables the regulatory agency to have an oversight of clinical trials with investigational medicinal products. Once registered, the EudraCT number can be entered in the ethics application and the EudraCT forms can be printed out for clinical trial authorisation (CTA) from the MHRA.

The ethics application form can be downloaded or accessed online from the COREC website. The researcher should put his or her application through the central allocation system with an appropriate REC if the proposed project is a clinical trial of investigational medicinal products (CTIMP), or is likely to take place in more than one domain. For non-CTIMP trials that are conducted within one domain, the researcher has the option of approaching the local research ethics committee directly. A domain is an area covered by a strategic health authority (England), a health board (Scotland), a regional office of the NHS Wales Department or the whole of Northern Ireland. Once a validation letter is received by the chief investigator from the main REC, a site-specific assessment for the suitability of the investigation, site and facilities may be submitted to a relevant REC by the principal investigator.

Types of paediatric clinical trials

Researchers need to justify the need to conduct the study concerned. The need of the investigation should be weighed against the prevalence of the condition to be treated, the seriousness of the condition, the availability of alternative treatments, the novelty of the compound, uniqueness of the conditions in paediatrics, the age ranges of the children, unique safety concerns in paediatrics and the unique require-ment of paediatric formulations that serve the needs of the population.

Paediatric formulation

The lack of suitable formulations in paediatrics has been highlighted by various authors in various countries ('t Jong *et al.*, 2004; Chui *et al.*, 2005; Nunn and Williams, 2005). The suitability includes palatability, appropriate strength and dose volume, favour and colours and route. Young children cannot swallow tablets, and liquids, suspensions, chewable tablets and suppositories may be needed for children of different age groups.

The concentrations of licensed medications may be too high, necessitating further manipulation in the form of dilution with an excipient. However, when the concentration is low, the dose volume may be too large for some children. The excipients in many liquid formulations may not be suitable for selected patient groups. For example, the propylene glycol content in amprenavir liquid formulation makes it unsuitable for children under 4 years of age. Severe delayed-onset hypersensitivity reaction was associated with formulation of amoxicillin liquid; the reaction may have been caused by the exicipent (Chopra *et al.*, 1989). Sweeteners, dyes and other excipients may cause adverse reactions and should be identified and restricted in paediatric formulations (Kumar *et al.*, 1996). Some clinical studies have been directed to ascertain the effect of drug concentration and frequency of administration on target organs. For example, in one study mercapt-amine drops 0.11% and 0.3% were administered at hourly and 6-hourly intervals, respectively, to ascertain whether a high concentration would reduce the need for frequent administration of the eye drops (MacDonald et al., 1990).

Pharmacokinetic study

Pharmacokinetic studies are performed to support formulation develop-ments and to determine pharmacokinetic parameters in different age groups to support dosing recommendations (E11) (ICH, 2000). They are generally conducted in children with a disease, which may lead to higher inter-individual variability than in adult health volunteers, although the data reflect clinical use better.

Single-dose pharmacokinetic studies may provide sufficient infor-mation for dosage selection in medicinal product that exhibit linear pharmacokinetics. Medicinal products that exhibit non-linearity in absorption, distribution and elimination may require steady-state studies. Such an approach has been used to assess the pharmacokinetics of an extemporaneously prepared sotalol syrup formulation in neonates, infants, and younger and older children. Scheduled blood samples were taken over a 36-hour time interval following dose administration (Saul et al., 2001).

Children are not usually subject to dose escalation studies similar to those carried out in adult populations; an extrapolation approach has been proposed to estimate paediatric dosages (Johnson, 2005). The use of such methods depends on the question to be answered, the availability of patients, and the practical and ethical problems in obtaining blood samples.

The use of population pharmacokinetics and a sparse sampling approach allow each patients to contribute as few as two to four observations at predetermined times to an overall population. Use of the area under the curve (AUC) will minimise the number of samples required from each patient. Population models allow researchers to assess and quantify potential sources of variability in exposure and response in the target population. Population pharmacokinetics seeks to discover which measurable pathophysiological factors cause changes in the dose–concentration relationship and to what degree, so that the appropriate dosage can be recommended. The pharmacokinetic–pharmacodynamic approach has been used to assess sotalol syrup formulations (Shi et al., 2001). Ten blood samples were taken from

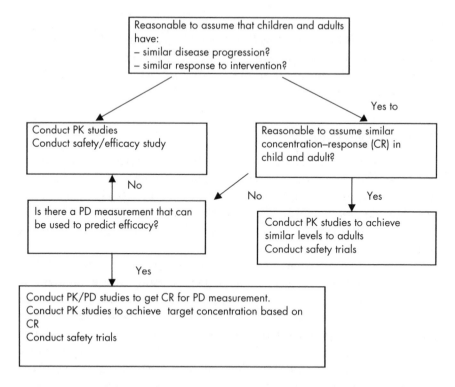

Figure 6.1 Paediatric study decision tree. PK, pharmacokinetics; PD, pharmacodynamics.

children with supraventricular or ventricular tachyarrhythmia following a single dose of sotalol, and doses were escalated over 3 days with an 8-hourly dosing. The data analysis used the NONMEM computer software program to obtain the population pharmacokinetic (PK) and pharmacodynamic (PD) parameter estimates.

A decision tree has been designed by the Center for Drug Evaluation and Research (CDER) at the Food and Drug Administration (Figure 6.1). Where there is similar disease progression and response to intervention and the PK/PD relationship of a drug is similar between adults and children, only PK studies and safety studies are recommended for bridging and dose determination.

Efficacy studies

When efficacy data from an adult study cannot be extrapolated to the targeted group of children, efficacy studies are required. This may necessitate developing, validating and employing different end-points for specific age groups. Study design for clinical trials has been covered elsewhere. The methodology for an efficacy study is similar to that in adult studies; what is different is the variety of presentations in children that are not found in adults.

Disodium pamidronate is licensed for use in Paget's disease and osteolytic lesions and bone pain in multiple myeloma and breast cancer in adults, but it has also been used in a variety of paediatric conditions: bone pain in Gaucher's disease (Ostlere *et al.*, 1991), osteogenesis imperfecta (Pizones *et al.*, 2005), mucolipidosis type III (Robinson *et al.*, 2002), McCune–Albright syndrome (Matarazzo *et al.*, 2002), malignant hypercalcaemia in childhood cancer (Kerdudo *et al.*, 2005) and juvenile spondyloarthropathies (Bukulmez and Colbert, 2002). Therefore a number of efficacy studies for disodium pamidronate are required to ascertain the efficacy for the disease concerned. The differences in the pathology of the diseases may require different dosage and administration regimens.

Research is needed to improve the delivery of drugs in children, either to enhance compliance via the route of choice or to identify alternative routes where the normal route of administration is unavailable or associated with severe side effects. The efficacy of administering ketamine and midazolam orally, rectally and intravenously to children receiving invasive procedures has been compared (Ozdemir *et al.*, 2004). It was found that the alternatives routes were equally effective. The use of other routes may mitigate the usual prolonged sedation and psychedelic effects of intravenous administration of ketamine/midazolam in children.

The quick onset and wearing off of sedation is advantageous in short procedures. For example, the intranasal and oral routes of midazolam have been compared (Lee-Kim *et al.*, 2004) and, although no difference in efficacy was found, the intranasal formulation had a quicker onset of action and a shorter duration of action than the oral preparation.

Occasionally, studies are carried out to target drugs direct to the site of action, thus reducing the exposure of other organs to the drugs. Oral and intravesical administrations of oxybutynin were compared in children with bladder dysfunction. The intravesical route produced a high plasma concentration, and was well tolerated and efficacious. A lack of significant systematic side effects observed in patients receiving oxybutynin via the intravesical route was attributed to the lack of metabolite commonly generated by the oral route. These studies demonstrate that the mode of administration affects the mechanism of action, side effects, pharmacokinetics and metabolism of oxybutynin (Massad *et al.*, 1992; Amark *et al.*, 1998).

Safety studies

Age-appropriate, normal laboratory values and clinical measurements should be used in adverse event reporting. Children with developing systems may respond differently to mature adults; some adverse events and drug interactions that occur in children may not be identified in adult studies. The effects of medicinal products on long-term growth and development may not be apparent, therefore long-term surveillance data may be needed to ascertain possible effects. Many established treatments in paediatrics have been conducted for a number of years, and the efficacy of such treatments has never been in doubt in the expert's mind. The use of morphine in neonate analgesia, for example, is a well-established treatment and no one would doubt that the drug does not work in such patient groups. Similarly, drugs such as sodium benzoate and phenylbutyrate have been used for more than 25 years for urea cycle defects, and diazoxide and chlorothiazide combination is a standard regimen for hyperinsulinism in neonates.

On the other hand, certain drugs have gone through the fast-track process and, at the time of authorisation, information on the safety of these medications has been limited, especially for children. In such cases non-interventional observations such as cohort or case–control studies could be a valuable tool to evaluate adverse events.

Safety studies fall into three categories, designed to demonstrate safety, detect new safety issues and evaluate known safety issues.

Cohort study

A cohort study is a prospective analysis of a population with a particular disease. Participants who are exposed to the study drug and those who are not on treatment are followed for a period of time and observed for development of the disease or result. Information on exposure is known throughout the follow-up period for each patient. The classic example is the use of anthracycline in childhood cancer. A long-term, non-interventional, observational follow-up of 607 children has shown that 5% of patients develop clinical cardiac failure 15 years after treatment. The risk increases with the increase in cumulative doses (Kremer *et al.*, 2001). Once a treatment is associated with certain toxicities, researchers can look at ways to minimise the effect. The relationship between the cardiotoxicity of anthracycline and its method of administration has been carried out in 44 children (Gupta *et al.*, 2003). A mean of 7 years after the end of therapy, there were no statistically significant differences between those receiving bolus injections and those receiving infusions.

A patient might be exposed to a drug at one time point but not at another. This is particularly important for metabolic diseases, where the progression of the disease should be monitored over a long period and patients should be monitored pre- and post-treatment. Incidence rates can be calculated from the population exposure. Cohort studies are useful when there is a need to know the incidence rates of adverse events in addition to the relative risks of adverse events.

Bias may be introduced into cohort studies when there is a loss to follow-up or when comparator groups are not well matched for potentially confounding factors. When sufficient numbers of patients exist, the data can be stratified to target a specific population. Cohort studies can be perceived as more ethically acceptable than placebo-controlled clinical trials, since a potentially beneficial treatment is not withheld from the participants, and cohort studies can be less expensive to conduct than randomised controlled trials. A longitudinal study is a cohort study with only one group, called the 'inception cohort'. Longitudinal studies are useful for following individuals with chronic diseases. Cohort studies can take a long time to complete when targeting rare diseases or diseases that take a long time to manifest.

Case–control studies

A case–control study is a retrospective analysis; it is generally easier to administer than a cohort study. Cases of diseases or events are identified. Controls and patients exposed to the treatment are selected from the source population. The exposure status of the two groups is compared using the odds ratio, an estimate of relative risk of exposure and non-exposure. Case–control studies are less expensive than cohort studies, but provide weaker empirical evidence than well-executed cohort studies. These studies are useful for identifying the relationship between drug treatments with one specific rare adverse event, or for identifying risk factors for adverse events. Risk factors can include renal and hepatic insufficiency that might modify the risk profile.

In a nested case–control study control sampling is density based; the control series represents the person–time distribution series in the source population. This means that the data about the cases and controls used in the study are nested within, or taken from, a cohort study. A cohort study collects data from every single individual from a predefined cohort with similar characteristics such as sex or year of birth. On top of that nested case–control study the control matches the duration of cohort membership within a certain time period. The control is randomly selected from the cohort, to a fixed multiple (e.g. 20 controls for each case). This methodology has been used recently to measure the risk of fatal and non-fatal self-harm in patients with first-episode depression receiving selective serotonin uptake inhibitors (SSRIs) and tricyclic antidepressants (Martinez et al., 2005).

Case–control studies are best for studying rare adverse events that take a long time to develop. A disadvantage of this type of study is that it is based on memory and recall, which can be biased, as well as on medical records, which can be incomplete.

Trial designs for rare diseases

Clinical trials should be scientifically sound. Any trial that may not test the underlying hypotheses are unethical and may expose the patients to the risk and burdens without yielding any meaningful results (Altman, 1980; Freeman, 1987b). Randomised, placebo-controlled clinical trials provide the best study result with the least number of patients. When calculating the sample size, the investigator takes into account the expected variability of the outcomes and the chosen probability of type I error. Clinical trials for rare diseases may require a long enrolment period to achieve a sufficiently large sample size to produce meaningful results.

Rare diseases with a frequency of 1 in 10 000 will require 600 participants on each arm to demonstrate an intervention that would reduce the mortality rate from 40% to 30% with a p value of 0.05. A sample size of 12 million would be required to produce 600 participants (Lilford et al., 1995). A long enrolment period is either impractical or meaningless because new procedures, new agents, improved diagnoses and better understanding of the disease may be developed during the intervening period. A clinical trial of itraconazole for the prevention of chronic granulomatous disease, for example, took 10 years to enroll just 39 patients (Gallin et al., 2003). Alternative approaches such as open protocol, open label, crossover designs and meta-analyses have been used to overcome the shortcomings of traditional design.

Open protocol design

Open protocol design has been used in the investigation of mercaptamine for nephropathic cystinosis and sodium phenylbutyrate for urea cycle defects. All eligible patients were given the drugs. The two drugs had been approved as orphan products in the USA. The evaluation of the data was difficult and included ancedotal evidence. As many patients were already on the drug, it was very difficult to conduct any other type of study.

Open label trials

Unlike the open protocol design, open label trials can be controlled. The greatest limitation of open trials is the lack of standard features of clinical trials such as placebo controls, randomisation and blinding of raters. Difficulty still remains in the evaluation of the efficacy of the drug, but they do provide important information regarding the safety use of drugs.

Historical control

Patients with rare, life-threatening diseases have limited life expectancy, and the use of placebo-controlled studies may be seen by such patients as unethical because they may be withheld from a possible cure. The use of historical controls can circumvent the issues of lack of sample size and the use of placebo. However, interpreting the result of such studies may be difficult. The absence of a placebo control group and factors affecting placebo treatment response often do not remain static over time, making comparisons of recent studies with earlier studies problematic. Historical control trials may take longer, because end-points are controlled against what is historically known. The disease must be well differentiated, with steady and rapid progress.

Bayesian designed trials

Bayesian designed trials provide probabilities of treatment effects that apply directly to the next patient who is similar to those treated in any completed or ongoing trial. This approach provides probabilities that can be used in formal decision analysis.

These probabilities are calculated on the basis of the observed data and a prior distribution of probabilities. The results of many small trials are insignificant, and many will say that the treatment is still unproven. However, any small improvement will bring prior equipoised belief in the direction of benefit. One could argue that a decision taken from a posterior belief that incorporates evidence from a randomised controlled trial, however insignificant, is more likely to be correct than a decision based simply on a prior belief with no evidence to support it (Lilford, 1995).

The design could reduce time and cost, providing greater incentives for pharmaceutical and biotechnology companies to become involved. And with more experimental therapies to be tried, more people will be able to participate in clinical trials in the future.

Whenever a patient's response can be evaluated before the enrolment of subsequent patients, different designs can be used. In the 'play the winner' design, a participant is assigned to one treatment and if the outcome is successful then the next participant is assigned to the same treatment (Zelen, 1969). On the other hand, if the treatment is a failure, the next participant will be treated with another treatment. The limitation is that the response may be delayed or may not be available when the next participant arrives.

Crossover design

Crossover design may help to reduce the sample size while providing enough power to validate the result. Patients receive the two study treatments sequentially and are evaluated for a response after each treatment. Provided that there is no period of carryover effects and dropouts, crossover studies can match the power of traditional designs. However, the validity of this design is based on the assumptions mentioned above that are relatively difficult to achieve in a clinical setting. The treatment effect must be realised immediately after it is initiated and lost immediately on cessation. This condition may be fulfilled in short-acting compounds such as cytokines but not in long-acting compounds such as the use of Lorenzo oil in adrenaleukodystophy. Similarly the end-points must be clearly defined and measurable, and the symptoms must manifest in a short latency period. Otherwise they could occur after cessation of one treatment and after the next treatment is commenced.

Another limitation of the crossover design is the lack of long-term safety data. Patients switch from one therapy to another and the evaluation period tends to be short. The use of such a design may be more equitable to research participants. Every participant will have a chance to receive the new treatment, whereas, in the traditional design, only half the patients actually receive it.

Surrogate end-point

Surrogate end-points may be used in rare diseases where the study of the true end-point is impossible. A surrogate end-point or marker is a laboratory measurement or physical sign that is used in therapeutic trials as a substitute for a clinically meaningful end-point that measures directly how a patient feels, functions or survives. Changes induced by a therapy on a surrogate end-point are expected to reflect changes in a clinically meaningful end-point. The changes in surrogate response variables are likely to occur before a clinical event, so less time is needed for a trial. A surrogate end-point can be a legal basis for drug approval in many countries.

For life-threatening diseases, the speed in determining the benefit effect of a treatment is crucial. Surrogate end-points such as CD4 count and viral load are routinely used as markers for antiretroviral treatment. Similarly, in Gaucher's disease, ferritin is a marker for disease progression. However, in some patients, the association between the surrogate marker and disease progression might not be apparent. In orphan drug studies using Lorenzo oil for adrenoleukodystrophy, the reduction in serum long-chain fatty acids is not closely associated with a reduction in disease progress. A surrogate end-point must be validated (Prentice, 1989). For a surrogate end-point to be an effective substitute for clinical outcome, the effects of the intervention on the surrogate must reliably predict the overall effect on the clinical outcome (i.e there should be a strong, independent, consistent association between the surrogate end-point and the clinical end-point).

Some workers have suggested that the use of a surrogate end-point as a sole determinant of efficacy should be used only in phase II studies (Fleming and DeMets, 1996). The surrogate end-points in some incidences do not predict the true clinical effects of interventions. This is because a surrogate end-point might not involve the same pathophysiological process that results in the clinical outcome. Even when it does, some disease pathways are probably causally related to the clinical outcome and not related to the surrogate end-point. The most plausible explanation is usually that the intervention has unintended mechanisms of action that are independent of the disease process.

Researchers need to ensure that the cost savings for not measuring clinical events is not negated by the cost for extra equipment and tests for surrogate markers. They also need to consider whether the result generated is acceptable to scientific and regulatory communities and the safety data are sufficient from a smaller sample size.

Underpowered studies

Meta-analysis may make small studies meaningful by providing a means to combine the results with those of other similar studies to enable estimates of an intervention's efficacy. Small trials may not be able to test a hypothesis, but they may provide valuable information of treatment effects using confidence intervals (Edwards *et al.*, 1997). Similarly, others argue that a sample size that results in a *p* value of 0.1 can be informative and decisions have to be made; even where there is no trial evidence, a little unbiased evidence is better than none. A study might have only limited ability to detect an effect, but participants should be allowed to make an autonomous decision.

Some argue that meta-analysis is meaningful only when researchers explicitly plan the study such that a prospective meta-analysis is possible. Research carries burdens in addition to those encountered in clinical context, such as extra follow-up visits, investigations and discomforts. These burdens cannot be justified by potential benefits to participants, but only by their ability to increase the value of the knowledge to be gained.

The general criticism of alternative trial designs is that the confidence intervals for the estimate of the magnitude of the treatment effect may be wide. The counter-argument is that, when traditionally powered studies fail to produce definite results, the new treatment can still be adopted and additional long-term safety and efficacy data might be gained (Lagakos, 2003).

At a logistic level, the prevalence of rare diseases and the geographical dispersion of such patients have made multicentre studies unavoidable. The investigation of botulism immunoglobulin involved 59 study sites and 120 patients (Haffner, 1998). The enormity of coordinating a trial of such scale is a challenge to many investigator-led researches. The requirement for a single sponsor that is responsible for multinational, multicentre trials, as stipulated by the EU Directive, provides another hindrance.

References

Altman D G (1980). Statistics and ethics in medical research III: how large a sample? *BMJ* 281: 1336–1338.

Amark P, Eksborg S, Juneskans O, *et al.* (1998). Pharmacokinetics and effects of intravesical oxybutynin on the paediatric neurogenic bladder. *Br J Urol* 82: 859–864.

Autret E, Dutertre J P, Barbier P, *et al.* (1993). Parental opinions about biomedical research in children in Tours, France. *Des Pharmacol Ther* 20: 64–71.

Barfield R C, Church C (2005). Informed consent in pediatric clinical trials. *Curr Opin Pediatr* 17: 20–24.

Beauchamp T L, Childress J F (2001). *Principles of Biomedical Ethics.* New York: Oxford University Press.

Belmont Report (1978) Ethical Principles and Guidelines for the Protection of Human Subjects of Research, National Commission for the Protection of Human Subjects of Biomedical and Behavioral Research. DHEW Publication OS 78-0012.

Brocklehurst P (1994). Randomised controlled trials in perinatal medicine. 2 Recruitment of a pregnant woman or her newborn child into more than one trial. *Br J Obstet Gynaecol* 104: 765–767.

Bukulmez H, Colbert R A (2002). Juvenile spondyloarthropathies and related arthritis. *Curr Opin Rheumatol* 14: 531–535.

Burgess E, Singhal N, Amin H, *et al.* (2003). Consent for clinical research in the neonatal intensive care unit, a retrospective survey and a prospective study. *Arch Dis Child Fetal Neonatal Ed* 88: F321–F323.

COREC (Central Office for Research Ethics Committees) (2006). Guidelines for researches: patient information sheet and consent form. http://www.corec. org.uk (accessed 13 August 2006).

Chopra R, Roberts J, Warrington R J (1989). Severe delayed-onset hypersensitivity reactions to amoxicillin in children. *Can Med Assoc J* 140: 921–923.

Chui J, Tordoff J, Reith D (2005). Changes in availability of paediatric medicines in Australia between 1998 and 2002. *Br J Clin Pharmacol* 59: 736–742.

Corbie-Smith G, Thomas S B, Williams M V, *et al.* (1999). Attitudes and beliefs of African Americans toward participation in medical research. *J Gen Intern Med* 14: 537–546.

Department of Health (2005). *Research Governance Framework for Health and Social Care.* http://www.dh.gov.uk/assetRoot/04/12/24/27/04122427.pdf (accessed 13 August 2006).

Edwards S J L, Lifford R J, Braunholtz D A, *et al.* (1997). Why 'underpowered' trials are not necessarily unethical. *Lancet* 350: 804–807.

Edwards S B, Lifford R J, Braunholtz D A, *et al.* (1998). Ethical issues in the design and conduct of randomised controlled trial. *Health Technol Assess* 2: 1–132.

Ellis P M, Dowett SM, Butow P N, *et al.* (1999). Attitudes to randomised clinical trials amongst out-patients attending medical oncology clinic. *Health Expect* 2: 33–43.

Fleming T R, DeMets D L (1996). Surrogate end points in clinical trials. Are we being misled? *Ann Intern Med* 125: 605–613.

Flory J, Emanuel F (2004). Interventions to improve research participants' understanding in informed consent for research, a systematic review. *JAMA* 292: 1593–1601.

Freedman B (1987a). Equipoise and the ethics of clinical research. *N Engl J Med* 317: 141–145.

Freedman B (1987b). Scientific value and validity as ethical requirements for research: a proposed explication. *IRB Rev Hum Subjects Res* 9: 7–10.

Forrow I, Taylor W, Arnold R (1992). Absolutely relative: how research results are summarised can affect treatment decision. *Am J Med* 92: 121–124.

Gallin J I, Alling D W, Malech H L, *et al.* (2003). Itraconazole to prevent fungal infections in chronic granulomatous disease. *N Engl J Med* 348: 2416–2422.

Gillick v West Norfolk AHA [1985] 3 All ER 402, at 423–4. http://adc.bmjjournals.com/cgi/content/full/archdischild%3B82/2/177?maxtoshow=%3Feaf#title (accessed 8 May 2006).

Gupta M, Steinherz P G, Cheung N K, *et al.* (2003). Late cardiotoxicity after bolus versus infusion anthracycline therapy for childhood cancers. *Med Pediatr Oncol* 40: 343–347.

Haffner M E (1998). Designing clinical trials to study rare disease treatment. *Drug Info J* 32: 957–960.

Harth S C, Thong Y H (1990). Socioeconomic and motivational characteristics of parents who volunteer their children for clinical research: a controlled study. *BMJ* 300: 1372–1375.

Hewlett S (1996). Consent to clinical research – adequately voluntary or substantially influenced? *J Med Ethics* 22: 232–237.

Hoehn K S, Wernovsky, Rychik J, *et al.* (2005). What factors are important to parents making decisions about neonatal research? *Arch Dis Child Fetal Neonatal Ed* 90: F267–269.

International Conference on Harmonisation (ICH) (1996) E6(R1): Good Clinical Practice: Consolidated Guideline. www.ich.org (accessed 9 August 2006).

ICH (2000) E11: Clinical Investigation of Medicinal Products in the Paediatric Population. www.ich.org (accessed 9 August 2006).

Johnson T N (2005) Modelling approaches to dose estimation in children. *Br J Clin Pharmacol* 59: 663–669.

Kerdudo C, Aerts I, Fattet S, *et al.* (2005). Hypercalcemia and childhood cancer: a 7-year experience. *J Pediatr Hematol Oncol* 27: 23–27.

Kodish E (2003). Pediatric ethics and early-phase childhood cancer research: conflicted goals and the prospect of benefit. *Account Res* 10: 17–25.

Kremer L C, van Dalen E C, Offirnga M, *et al.* (2001). Anthracycline-induced clinical heart failure in a cohort of 607 children: long-term follow-up study. *J Clin Oncol* 19: 191–196.

Kumar A, Aitas A T, Hunter A G, *et al.* (1996). Sweeteners, dyes, and other excipients in vitamin and mineral preparations. *Clin Pediatr (Philadelphia)* 35: 443–450

Kupst M J, Patenaude A F, Walco G A, *et al.* (2003). Clinical trials in paediatric cancer: parental perspective on informed consent. *Pediatr Hematol Oncol* 25: 787–790.

Lagakos S W (2003). Clinical trials and rare disease. *N Engl J Med* 348: 2455–2456.

Langley J M, Halperin S A, Mills E L, *et al.* (1998). Parental willingness to enter a child in a controlled vaccine trial. *Clin Invest Med* 21: 12–16.

Lantos J D (1999). The 'inclusion effect' in clinical trials. *J Paediatr* 134: 130–131

Lavori P W, Sugaman J, Hays M T, *et al.* (1999). Improving informed consent in clinical trials: a duty to experiment. *Control Clin Trials* 20: 187–193.

Lee-Kim S J, Fadavi S, Punwani I, *et al.* (2004). Nasal versus oral midazolam sedation for pediatric dental patients. *J Dent Child* 71: 126–130.

Lilford R J, Thornton J G, Braunholtz D (1995). Clinical trials and rare diseases: a way out of a conundrum. *BMJ* 311: 1621–1625.

MacDonald I M, Noel L P, Mintsioulis G, *et al.* (1990). The effect of topical cysteamine drops on reducing crystal formation within the cornea of patients affected by nephropathic cystinosis. *J Pediatr Ophthalmol Strabismus* 27: 272–274.

Manning D J (2000). Presumed consent in emergency neonatal research. *J Med Ethics* 26: 249–253.

Martinez C, Riethbrock S, Wise L, *et al.* (2005). Antidepressant treatment and the risk of fatal and non-fatal self harm in first episode depression: nested case-control study. *BMJ* 330: 389–395.

Mason S (1997). Obtaining informed consent for neonatal randomised controlled trials – an 'elaborate ritual'? *Arch Dis Child* 77: F143–145.

Mason S A, Allmark P J (2000). Obtaining informed consent to neonatal randomised controlled trials, interviews with parents and clinicians in the Euricon study. *Lancet* 356: 2045–2051.

Massad C A, Kogan B A, Trigo-Rocha F E (1992). The pharmacokinetics of intra-vesical and oral oxybutynin chloride. *J Urol* 148: 595–597.

Matarazzo P, Lala R, Masi G, *et al.* (2002). Pamidronate treatment in bone fibrous dysplasia in children and adolescents with McCune-Albright syndrome. *J Pediatr Endocrinol Metab* 15(suppl 3): 929–937.

MHRA (Medicines and Healthcare products Regulatory Agency) (2006). Algorithm. http://www.mhra.gov.uk/home/idcplg?IdcService=GET_FILE&dDocName=con009394&RevisionSelectionMethod=Latest (accessed 13 August 2006).

Modi N (1994). Clinical trials and neonatal intensive care. *Arch Dis Child* 70: F231–F232.

Morley C J (1997). Consent is not always practical in emergency treatments. *BMJ* 314: 1480.

Morley C J, Lau R, Davis P G, Morse C (2005). What do parents think about enrolling their premature babies in several research studies? *Arch Dis Child Fet Neonatal Ed* 90: F225–F228.

Nunn T, Williams J (2005). Formulation of medicines for children. *Br J Clin Pharmacol* 59: 674–676.

Ostlere L, Warner T, Meunier P J, *et al.* (1991). Treatment of type 1 Gaucher's disease affecting bone with aminohydroxypropylidene bisphosphonate. *Q J Med* 79: 503–515.

Ozdemir D, Kayserili E, Arslanoglu S, *et al.* (2004). Ketamine and midazolam for invasive procedures in children with malignancy: a comparison of routes of intravenous, oral, and rectal administration. *J Trop Pediatr* 50: 224–228.

Pizones J, Plotkin H, Parra-Garcia J L, *et al.* (2005). Bone healing in children with osteogenesis imperfecta treated with bisphosphonates. *J Pediatr Orthop* 25: 332–335.

Prentice R L (1989). Surrogate endpoints in clinical trials: definition and operational criteria. *Stat Med* 8: 431–440.

Robinson C, Baker N, Noble J, *et al.* (2002). The osteodystrophy of mucolipidosis type III and the effects of intravenous pamidronate treatment. *J Inherit Metab Dis* 25: 681–693.

Rogers C G, Tyson J E, Kennedy K A, *et al.* (1998). Conventional consent with opting in versus simplified consent with opting out: an exploratory trial for studies that do not increase patient risk. *J Paediatr* 132: 606–611.

Rossi W C, Reynolds W, Nelson R M (2003). Child assent and parental permission in pediatric research. *Theor Med Bioeth* 24: 131–148.

Rothmier J D, Lasley Mand Shapiro G G (2003). Factors influencing parental consent in pediatric clinical research. *Pediatrics* 111: 1037–1041.

Royal College of Paediatrics and Child Health: Ethics Advisory Committee (2000). Guidelines for the ethical conduct of medical research involving children. *Arch Dis Child* 82: 177–182.

Saul J P, Schaffer M S, Karpawich P P, *et al.* (2001). Single-dose pharmacokinetics of sotalol in a pediatric population with supraventricular and/or ventricular tachyarrhythmia. *J Clin Pharmacol* 41: 35–43.

Schmidt B, Gille P, Caco C, *et al.* (1999). Do sick newborn infants benefit from participation in a randomised clinical trial? *J Pediatr* 134: 151–155.

Schwartz L, Woloshin S, Black W, *et al.* (1997). The role of numeracy in understanding the benefit of screening mammography. *Ann Intern Med* 127: 966–972.

Shavers V, Burmeister L (2002). Racial differences in factors that influence the willingness to participate in medical research studies. *Ann Epidemiol* 12: 248–256.

Shi J, Ludden T M, Melikian A P, *et al.* (2001). Population pharmacokinetics and pharmacodynamics of sotalol in pediatric patients with supraventricular or ventricular tachyarrhythmia. *J Pharmacokinet Pharmacodyn* 28: 555–575.

Siminoff L A (2003). Toward improving the informed consent process in research with humans. *IRB* 25(suppl 25): S1–3.

Smith R (2000). Babies and consent: yet another NHS scandal. *BMJ* 320: 1285–1286.

Snowdon C, Garcia J, Elbourne D (1997). Making sense of randomisation; response of parents of critically ill babies to random allocation of treatment in a clinical trial. *Soc Sci Med* 45: 1337–1355.

Stenson B J, Becher J C, McIntosh N (2004). Neonatal research: the parental perspective. *Arch Dis Child Fetal Neonatal Ed* 89: F321–F323.

't Jong G W, Eland I A, Sturkenboom M C, *et al.* (2004). Unlicensed and off-label prescription of respiratory drugs to children. *Eur Respir J* 23: 310–313.

Tait A R, Voepel-Lewis T, Siewert M, *et al.* (1998). Factors that influence parent's decisions to consent their child's participation in clinical anesthesia research. *Anesth Analg* 86: 50–53.

Tait A R, Voepel-Lewis T, Mallviya S (2003). Do they understand? Part I: parental consent for children participating in clinical anesthesia and surgery research. *Anesthesiology* 98: 603–608.

Tait A R, Voepel-Lewis T, Malviya S (2004). Factors that influence parents' assessments of the risks and benefits of research involving their children. *Pediatrics* 113: 727–732.

Tarnowski K J, Allen D M, Mayhall C, *et al.* (1990). Readability of paediatric biomedical research informed consent forms. *Pediatrics* 85: 58–62.

van Stuijvenberg M, Suur M H, de Vos S, *et al.* (1998). Informed consent, parental awareness, and reasons for participating in a randomised controlled study. *Arch Dis Child* 79: 120–125.

Waggoner W C, Mayo D M (1995). Who understands? A survey of 25 words or phrases commonly used in proposed clinical research consent forms. *IRB* 17: 6–9.

Zelen M (1969). Play the winner rule and the controlled clinical trial. *J Am Stat Assoc* 64: 131–146.

Zupancic J A, Gillie P, Streiner D L, *et al.* (1997). Determinants of parental authorisation for involvement of newborn infants in clinical trials. *Pediatrics* 99: 117.

Index